juiceman

Andrew Cooper

MICHAEL JOSEPH
an imprint of
PENGUIN BOOKS

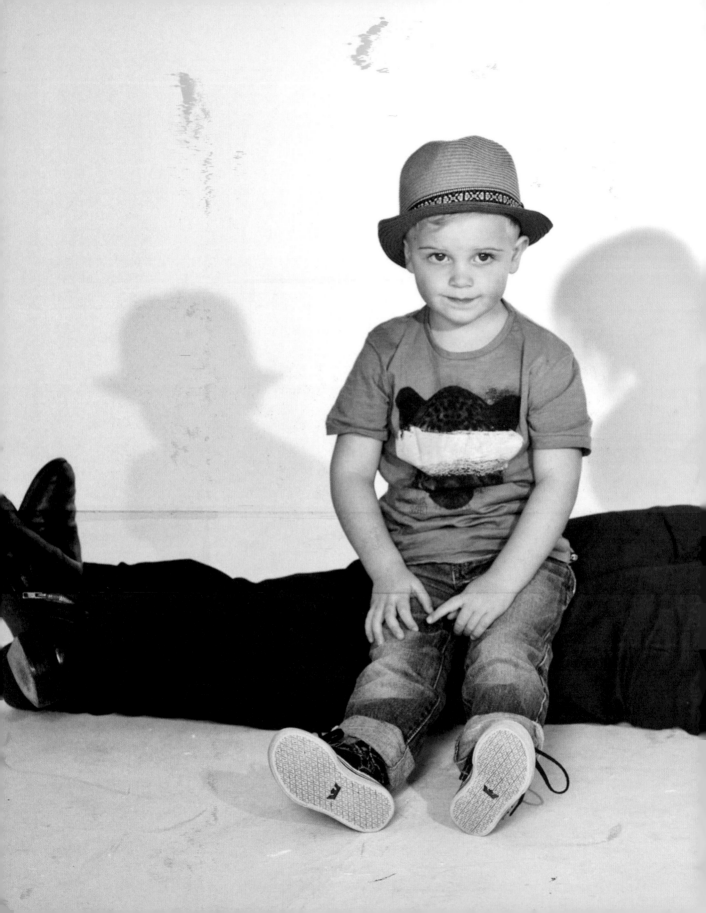

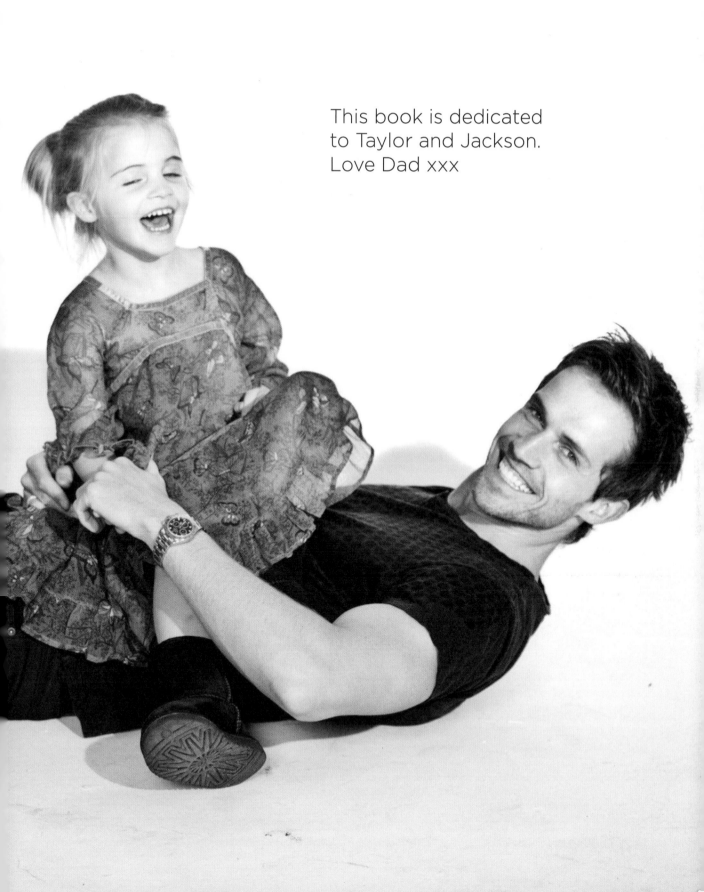

This book is dedicated
to Taylor and Jackson.
Love Dad xxx

CONTENTS

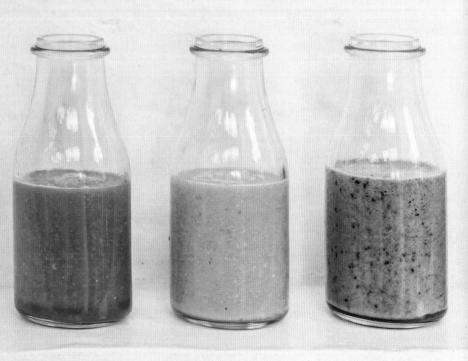

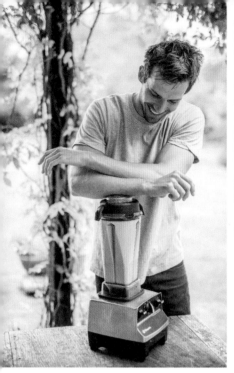
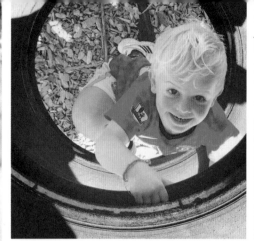
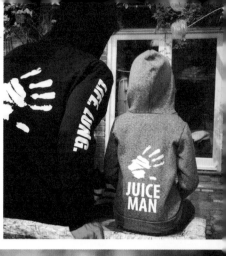
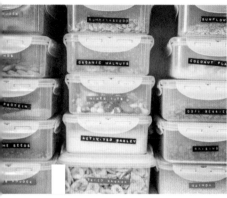
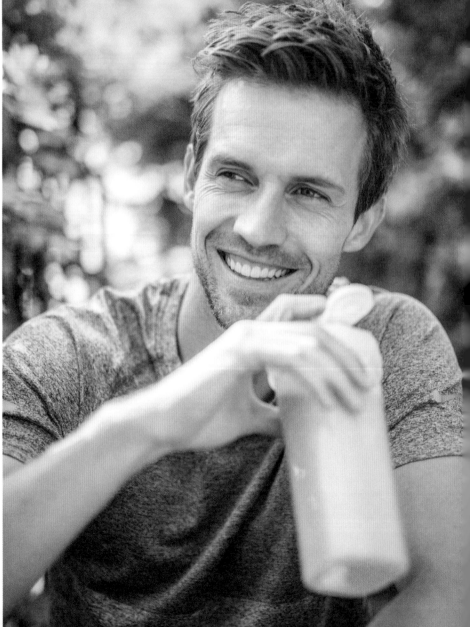
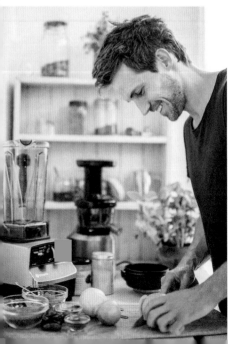

THE JUICEMAN STORY

As a northern lad growing up, writing a book about juice was never something I imagined I would do! My introduction to fresh fruit and vegetables did start at an early age as my mum made sure that we had as much home-grown and natural food as possible. But it wasn't until I was a bit older that I realized perhaps Mum actually does know best – even though some of the soups she made were a bit . . . odd. (Sorry, Mum.) Now I feel really lucky to have been raised in that way.

Some of my best memories are of home-cooked family meals. My granddad Andrew was a baker and my granddad Jack a butcher, so I was surrounded by enthusiastic food lovers from an early age. They taught me all about food: how to touch, smell and taste ingredients. And I've always been interested in where food comes from, having spent hours digging up potatoes and pulling up carrots for my mum on a Sunday morning.

When I was seventeen, I broke the family mould and headed to London to pursue a career in music and fashion. I was no different to anyone else my age and was over-doing it by going out all the time. But I managed to supplement my busy lifestyle with healthy food and juices. I bought my first juicer at nineteen, an old-fashioned model that you had to put a paper liner into to catch the pulp. All of my friends thought I was an oddball for buying it. But it made great juice, even though the washing-up afterwards was a killer.

Luckily juicers became increasingly efficient and my love for juicing grew and grew. I would take regular trips to the farmers market in Queens Park for the wonderful fresh fruit and veg. Then my wife Jane and I had our very own escape to the country when our daughter, Taylor, was born and we bought an old fruit farm up in Cheshire.

At the same time, I was flying to the US weekly for modelling and acting jobs. When being fit and healthy and looking as good as possible is part of your job, it really makes you think about what you are putting into your body. Plus kids, as anyone with them will know, add a whole new dimension to your life. I was experiencing tiredness that I never knew existed and so I decided to try to combat this by incorporating as many nutritious foods into my diet as possible. I found juicing to be a brilliant way to achieve this.

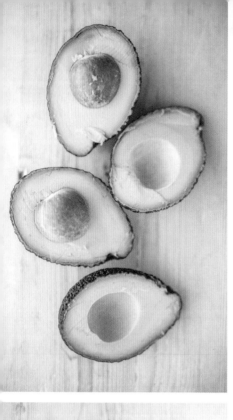
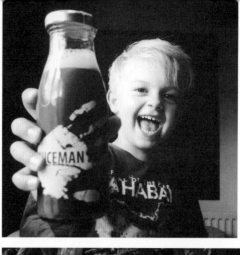
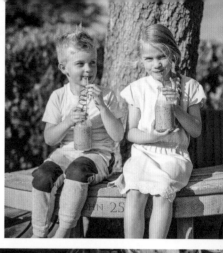
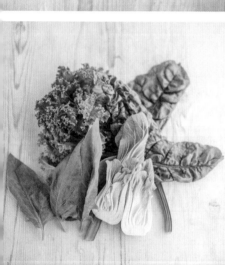
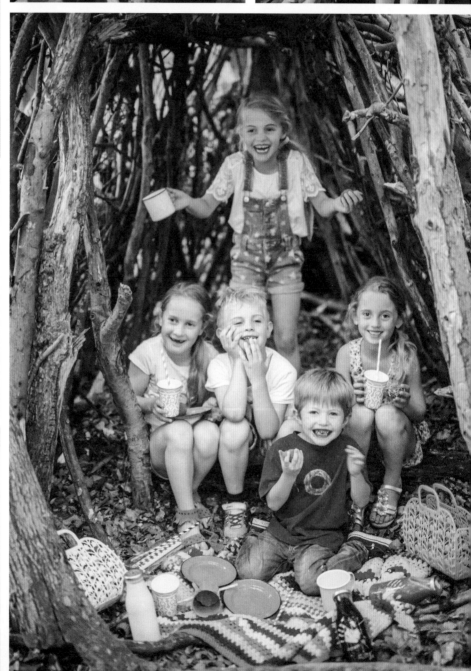
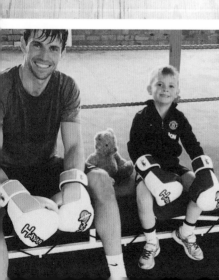

GET YOUR 5-A-DAY IN A GLASS

I believe that is no better way to load up on vitamins and enzymes than having a glass of green juice. At Juiceman, we can get 2 kilograms of veg into a 500ml bottle of juice. Imagine eating through 2 kilograms of veg on your plate! As for smoothies, they are my meal in a glass because my nutritional needs can be met in an instant. If I'm home late or I need a quick fix, I will always make a green smoothie.

Fruit and vegetables are simply amazing. The amount of vitamins and enzymes that they contain is unreal. When Jane and I moved back to London, one of the best things I did was plant my own veg patch – I couldn't believe how much I could grow in such a small area.

I'm a firm believer in the fresher the better. The difference between an apple picked from the tree to one from the supermarket is huge. To harness that freshness, or get as close to it as possible, was my ultimate goal. And by juicing the freshest produce, all the vitamins, enzymes and minerals can be in your system in an instant.

I started to share my enthusiasm for juices, smoothies and raw food with my family and friends. I became known as The Juiceman as I did home deliveries like a local milkman! As demand grew, my cold-pressed juice company was born.

LIFE. LONG.

My handprint is the logo used on all of our products and it symbolises the journey from seed to bottle. It emphasises my original vision to create an ethical and sustainable juice business and you will also see it used throughout this book to flag up my absolute favourite recipes (see page 12).

Unfortunately, we're now a society obsessed with fad diets and losing weight when what we really should be focusing on is our health. If we were all healthy, we wouldn't need to diet! The phrase 'Life. Long.' used on

Juiceman products sums up the Juiceman ethos: our wish for health and longevity. We believe that a nutritious diet can go a long way and it's our aim to make this a sustainable lifelong habit that is easy, fun and enjoyable.

And now I want to share my passion and lifestyle with you, and to show that it's easy to create great-tasting and nutritious food and drinks at home.

This book can help you to:
- increase your energy levels
- get clearer skin
- reduce your cholesterol
- build stronger, healthier bones
- boost your immune system
- eliminate sugar and caffeine cravings
- get better-quality sleep
- improve recovery from exercise
- improve productivity

JUICE KIDS

A huge reason for starting Juiceman was my mission to get kids to enjoy nutritious juices and smoothies and to stop consuming so many processed foods and fizzy drinks. My own kids love the recipes in this book. Of course there are times when they will want candyfloss over a fresh organic apple and carrot juice – they are kids after all! But it's about finding a balance. There are lots of fun ways to integrate healthy food and drink recipes into their lives – such as smoothie bowls, ice lollies, ice cream and flavoured ice cubes. Like any Dad, I've had to be inventive with ways of getting them to eat the good stuff. Get your kids experimenting. My little guy Jackson loves making smoothies and juices with me – most mornings he is chief juicer in our house.

FOR THE OCCASION

Throughout the book you will come across these symbols on the recipes:

 JUICEMAN LOVES

I have given this stamp to the recipes I especially love. There are certain recipes I just cannot live without. I hope you like them as much as I do.

 SPICE RATING

If a recipe has a chilli by it, then it has a certain amount of spice.
I have rated the recipes with 1, 2 or 3 chillies.
1 chilli = A little kick, but nothing too much to worry about.
2 chillies = Quite fiery.
3 chillies = Hot!

 LOW SUGAR

Everyone is different in terms of how much sugar they want or need in their diet. In this book, I use 'good' sugars from natural sources such as dates and coconut, but even so, they may not be suitable for everyone. I have a friend who is diabetic and can really only drink veg-based juices and smoothies. So if you have similar dietary requirements, watch out for this logo. These recipes are at least 90 per cent veg.

 COCKTAIL MIXER

There is a cocktail chapter in this book, but so many of the non-alcoholic recipes also make great cocktail mixers. So if you see this sign, feel free to try them with alcohol too.

 ENERGY

We often need an energy boost. For example, if planning a trip to the gym, it's important to make sure you are well fuelled and your energy levels are up. It's equally important to restock your energy stores post-workout. In my opinion there is no better way to do this than by drinking a power shake and eating a protein truffle (see p.91, p.92 and p.172). It's also important to ensure the right nutrition after your workout with good levels of carbohydrates and protein, which will help to aid muscle repair and make sure you get up the next day without aching or finding it too difficult to walk! Whatever your reason for needing an energy boost, if you see the Energy sign, this will be a good recipe for you.

 FAMILY

The recipes with the Family logo are the ones that everyone is sure to love – adults and kids alike. Try them out on your whole family and get everyone involved. These are so delicious that no one will believe how nutritious they are. Throw a handful of spinach into a strawberry smoothie and your kids won't know the difference. I love making smoothies with my kids and they drink some unbelievable concoctions. It feels good knowing that they're getting their 5-a-day goodness in a glass. You can then rest assured during a family night in with a family-size pizza! When my wife was pregnant with our son Jackson, she would drink green smoothies all the time. I'm convinced this is why he's such a healthy boy.

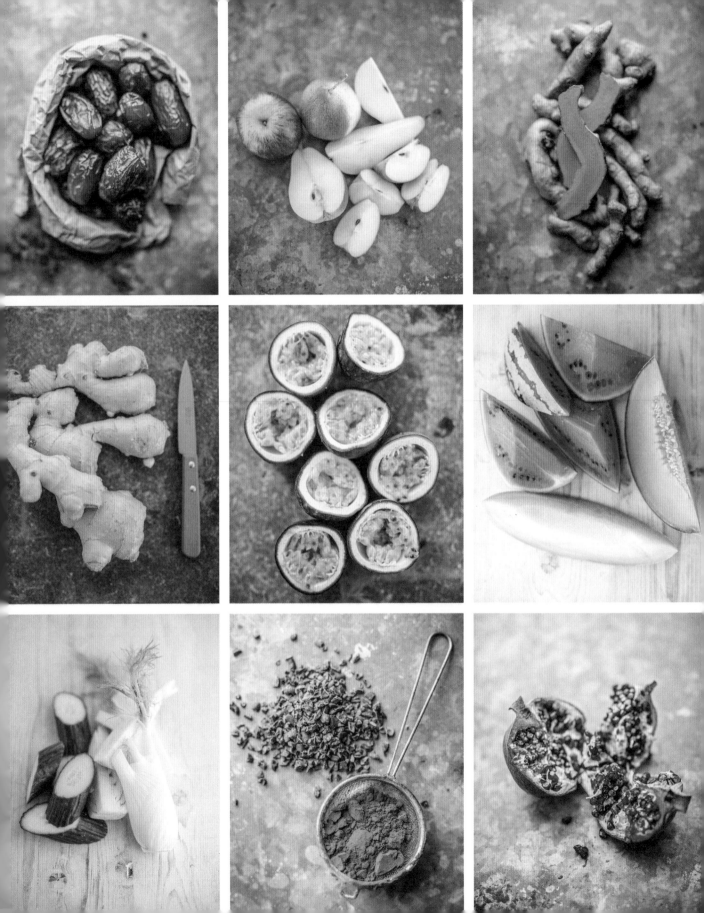

POWDERS

Spirulina: a blue-green algae that is considered a complete protein, boasting B-complex vitamins, beta-carotene, vitamin E, carotenoids, manganese, zinc, copper, iron, selenium and gamma-linolenic acid (GLA, an essential fatty acid). It is a great anti-inflammatory, good for immunity and brain boosting. Be warned that it has a strong flavour. I like to hide it in a blueberry or cacao smoothie.

Chlorella: a green algae in powder or tablet form that is protein rich. It is packed with chlorophyll, which makes it hugely detoxifying. It's high in omega-3 and many vitamins, especially A, B, C and E. It also contains 18 amino acids. I prefer it in tablet form and always take some with me when travelling.

Maca: this Peruvian root is my go-to for an energy boost and mood lift. It is also widely considered to help with both male and female sexual function by increasing libido and endurance. Overall, it is a great health-boosting supplement that is part of my daily regime. I take a minimum of one teaspoon per day in a smoothie.

Matcha: the most powerful form of green tea. Because it's ground and you therefore drink the whole leaf, Matcha has up to 137 times more antioxidants than regular green tea. It contains good levels of vitamin C, selenium, chromium, zinc and magnesium, and is rich in chlorophyll. I am a huge fan of Matcha in my green smoothies to kick-start the day.

Lucuma: a South American powder made from the fruit of the *Pouteria lucuma* tree. It is such a great addition to any smoothie as it provides 14 essential trace elements, including a considerable amount of potassium, sodium, calcium, magnesium and phosphorus.

SPORTS POWDERS:

Perm A vite: gut health is hugely important and this supplement helps to support a healthy digestive tract. I take it every morning on an empty stomach. It provides you with great levels of L-glutamine, MSM and contains slippery elm.

L-Glutamine: an essential supplement if you are heavily active and living a fast-paced lifestyle. I add a small scoop to my post-workout smoothie to aid recovery and increase fat burning. It's also another great supplement for your gut and digestion.

Hemp protein: hemp is the ultimate seed. Hemp protein powder is great because it is not only high in protein but also naturally contains 21 amino acids and BCAAs (branch chain amino acids). It is essentially the perfect recovery protein in a natural state. I add it to everything from shakes to smoothie bowls and cakes. My four-year-old son, Jackson, has pancakes and a chocolate milk-shake with a small scoop of hemp protein after his Saturday footie. Other natural protein powders to try are flax, rice and pea.

Activated whey: I prefer to take natural vegan protein most of the time, but I'm not adverse to pure whey. Activated whey is the purest version of whey protein and the best way to put on weight and bulk up due to the body's ability to absorb much higher amounts of the protein than it's natural state. I am also a fan of egg white protein for anyone looking to put on weight, as it is also high in amino acids and our bodies can easily process and utilize it.

MSM: a fantastic beauty supplement. MSM is an abbreviation for methyl-sulfonyl-methane, which is a natural sulphur compound. It improves joint flexibility and circulation while reducing stiffness, pain and swelling. It also increases the body's ability to flush out toxins and excess fluids. For all you ladies, listen up:

it produces generous quantities of collagen and keratin, which are amazing for hair, nails and skin!

EXOTIC INGREDIENTS:

Bee pollen: truly a golden substance. It is pretty much amazing in every way, from boosting the immune system to increasing energy and improving digestive health. I use it sparingly as it's such a luxury. It is important to know that it takes one bee one month, working eight hours a day, to produce one teaspoon of pollen. Each bee pollen pellet contains over two million flower pollen grains and one teaspoonful contains over 2.5 billion grains of flower pollen. Bee pollen is richer in protein than any animal source and contains more amino acids than beef, eggs or cheese of equal weight.

Colloidal silver: a great supplement to help fight everything from a common cold to flu and chest infections. It is also a great antiviral and anti-inflammatory, so can be taken orally or applied directly on the skin. I give this to my kids to boost their immunity when I suspect they may be coming down with something.

Chaga mushrooms: these typically grow on Birch trees and are considered the ultimate antioxidant. They are a true super-food and known to be hugely beneficial in boosting the immune system, and stabilizing blood pressure and cholesterol levels. Chaga has one of the highest antioxidant values of any food substance. If you compare the antioxidant capacity of chaga to blueberries, for example, it's pretty mind blowing: 36,557 to 24.5 (ORAC per 1g).

Reishi mushrooms: the king of medicinal mushrooms and called the 'mushrooms of immortality'. They are found growing on plum trees in the wild and were originally reserved for use only by royals. Their amazing benefits range from promoting a longer, healthier life,

to helping to prevent cancer and supporting liver regeneration and nerve growth.The powder form tastes a bit strange but I like to add it to my smoothies when I particularly need a health boost.

Deer antler extract: hugely beneficial in supporting recovery, and boosts endurance and strength, in training. It increases blood circulation, is an aphrodisiac and aids good sexual health. It is also known as a growth hormone so it will help you look and feel young.

Slippery elm: extracted from the bark of the slippery elm tree and hugely beneficial to all kinds of digestive issues from ulcers to colitis. The Cherokee used it as a salve to heal wounds due to its anti-inflammatory properties.

Yerba maté: Nearly everyone enjoys a cup of coffee. And we also know deep down that it is a slippery slope once you start drinking multiple cups daily. Yerba maté is a great way to get the energy and caffeine but without the addiction. It has also been associated with weight loss. I like to mix 50/50 with green tea and keep it in a flask to have as iced tea, or add it to smoothies.

Aloe vera: the gel is an amazing substance to aid healing and it is also great for your skin, whether eaten or used externally. It is great for supporting healthy digestion and detoxification and it's very alkalizing. Aloe vera contains many vitamins including A, C, E, folic acid, choline, B1, B2, B3 (niacin), B6 and B12. It also contains 20 minerals, including calcium, magnesium, zinc, chromium, selenium, sodium, iron, potassium, copper and manganese. To access the gel, lay the leaf down and firstly remove the sides. You will then need to remove each outer layer like you would fillet a fish. Throw the gel in a smoothie for a beauty boost.

EQUIPMENT

There is such a wide selection of gear available these days that you should be able to find the right kit to suit your budget and kitchen. Personally, I think it's worth investing in a good-quality juicer and blender, particularly if you're looking to use them every day. I try to assess the cost of things based on how much use I'll get out of them over time. I have had my Vitamix for five years and use it twice a day. In the same amount of time, I have probably gone through four toasters. If I spread out the cost of my Vitamix over just three years it comes out at £8.33 a month. All the other utensils can be bought pretty cheaply nowadays.

Here are the kitchen essentials you will need for this book and some suggestions of reliable brands:

- **Juicer:** Omega Vert, Breville, Philips, Hurom
- **Blender:** NutriBullet, Vitamix, Ninja
- **Knives**
- **Peeler**
- **Grater**
- **Chopping board**
- **Spatulas**
- **Teapot** for loose tea
- **Ice cube tray/lolly mould**
- **Glass Bottles or containers** for storage

So which juicer to use? There are two main types of juicer: centrifugal and masticating (cold press). Each has its advantages and disadvantages, so it's up to you really which one to go for. Here is the low-down on the two types:

Centrifugal juicers
- Generally cheaper.
- Work more quickly as they run at a higher rpm (rate per minute).
- The downside to a high rpm is that heat is released, which oxidizes the juice, reducing the shelf life.

- Not as effective as low-rpm juicers for juicing leafy greens.
- Yield is much lower than with a low-rpm juicer.
- A good entry-level option.

Masticating juicers
- Gives a better-quality juice as no oxidization occurs. Juices can be stored for up to 48 hours with minimal loss to the nutritional value.
- More efficient as these produce a higher yield.
- Often come with extra attachments to make nut butters, dips and sauces and even pasta.
- The low rpm means it's a much slower process.

The main thing to consider when deciding on your model and budget is that if you are investing with a view to use it daily, a more expensive juicer will give you far superior yield (juice content). With this in mind, you may end up out of pocket with a cheaper high-rpm juicer in the long run.

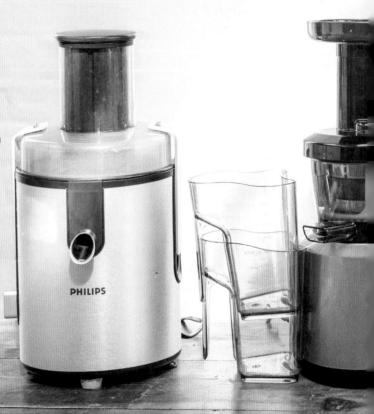

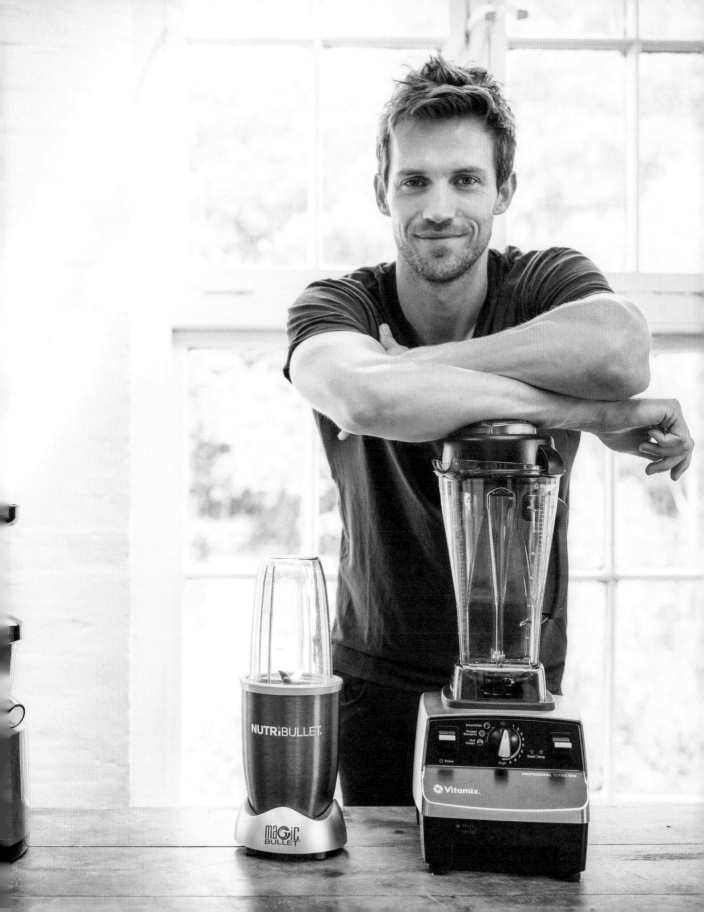

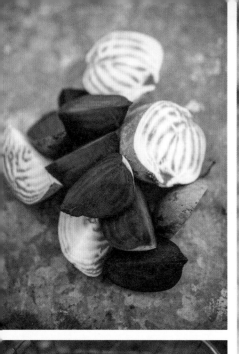

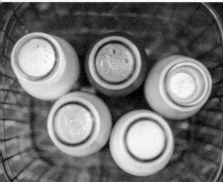

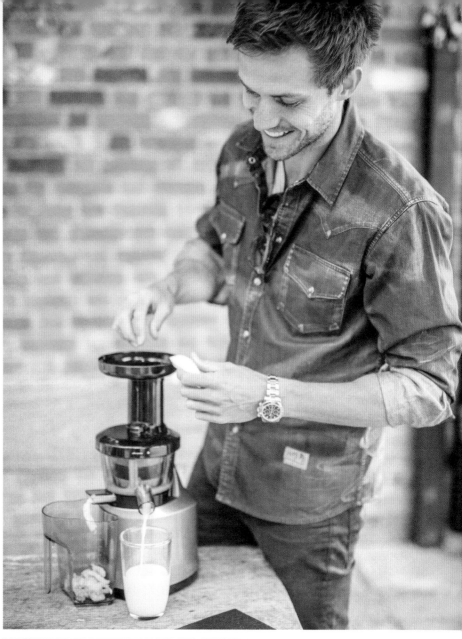

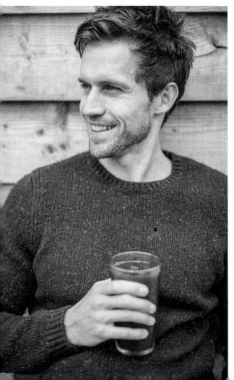

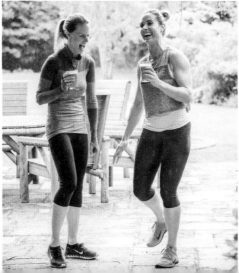

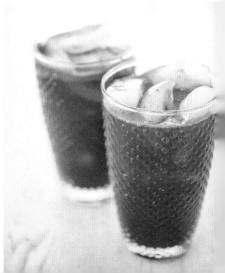

JUICES

I always get asked if I like juices or smoothies the best. The answer is simple – I like both! There are benefits to both, but what I like about juicing, is that by getting rid of the pulp you have a drink that your body can digest without any work. The amount of produce in one glass of juice means you can flood your body with a large amount of vitamins and enzymes. It would take most people all day to eat the amount of fruit and vegetables you can get in a glass of juice. In short, juices are a quick and easy way to help you stay fit and healthy.

Some of the biggest problems with juicing are the preparation, the washing up and figuring out where to put your cumbersome juicer. When buying a juicer make sure you pick the right one for your needs. Ideally find a space in your kitchen where your juicer and blender can sit. They need to be accessible. You could put some shelves above them and have your superfoods and ingredients there so they're always to hand.

The recipes in this chapter make around 400ml.

TOP TIPS

- Start off by juicing your citrus fruits.

- Always juice leafy veg and soft fruit in between root veg and hard fruit like apples.

- To keep your juicer easy to clean, pour a glass of water through at the end of your juicing session.

- Compost or reuse your pulp (see p.192–97).

All the recipes are for you to adapt and play with. If you love ginger, you can add it to almost any juice. Typically, all juices are specific in terms of nutritional value and have a base of colour and tone. But there are a number of ways you can add some extra zing, such as adding herbs and spices. Don't be afraid to experiment, tasting as you go.

The basic rule of thumb for juicing is juice what you like the taste of. To enjoy it and drink it, you have to like the taste. Your taste buds will probably change the more you juice. You may start off with carrot and orange and end up like me – a hardcore green juice drinker! At Juiceman, we spent six months testing out recipes to make sure they tasted amazing before putting them on sale. Even our straight vegetable juices are show-stoppingly good; it's all about the blend of flavours.

Certain ingredients go better together than others and the quantity you use of each ingredient obviously has a big effect on the taste. I have included a chart on page 13 to encourage you to improvise and try something new. Have a go and see where you end up!

Now let's get to the good stuff. You have all your kit and you are ready to go, so let's start making something . . .

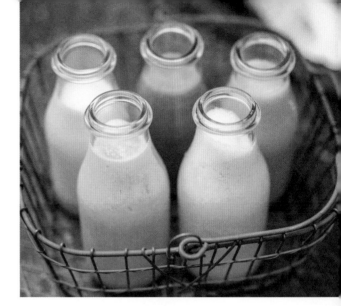

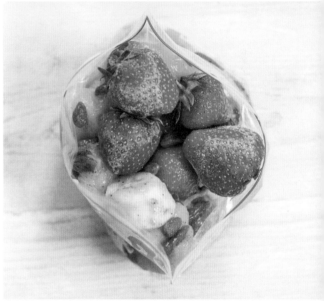

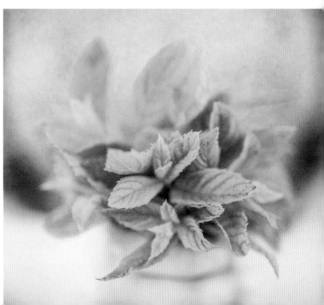

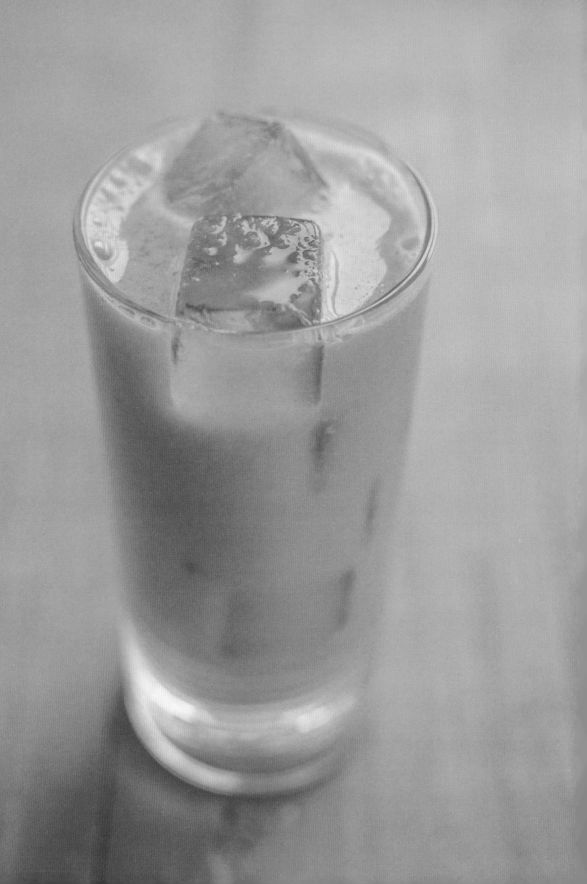

This is the best starter juice I know. Beautiful fresh carrots make a wonderful juice, and paired with apple and ginger they become irresistible. Ginger can vary in flavour and intensity – some varieties are much more fiery than others – so put in a little and add more depending on how you like it. I absolutely love it, so the hotter the better for me. For added vitality, throw in some freshly peeled turmeric root too.

THE ORIGINAL

1 apple

½ an orange, peeled

2.5cm piece of fresh root ginger, peeled

5 carrots

Wash all your ingredients and peel where instructed. Juice them one by one in the order they are listed and serve chilled or enjoy over ice.

JUICEMAN TIPS
Add a teaspoon of hemp oil for maximum vitamin A absorption. The ginger can be removed for kids. I juice the whole apple, including the core, but you can core it too.

JUICEMAN FACT
Carrots are the kings of vitamin A.

Summer is the season for watermelons. You'll be amazed at how much juice you can get out of one. It's also super hydrating and sweet but with minimal calories. Who needs slimline tonic when you have a watermelon about? My kids love this juice and it's perfect for when you're having your mates over for a BBQ.

WATERMELON COOLER

½ a lime, peeled

a small bunch of mint

½ a watermelon, peeled

Wash all your ingredients and peel where instructed. Juice them one by one in the order they are listed and serve chilled or enjoy over ice.

JUICEMAN FACT
Lime is a natural antibiotic.

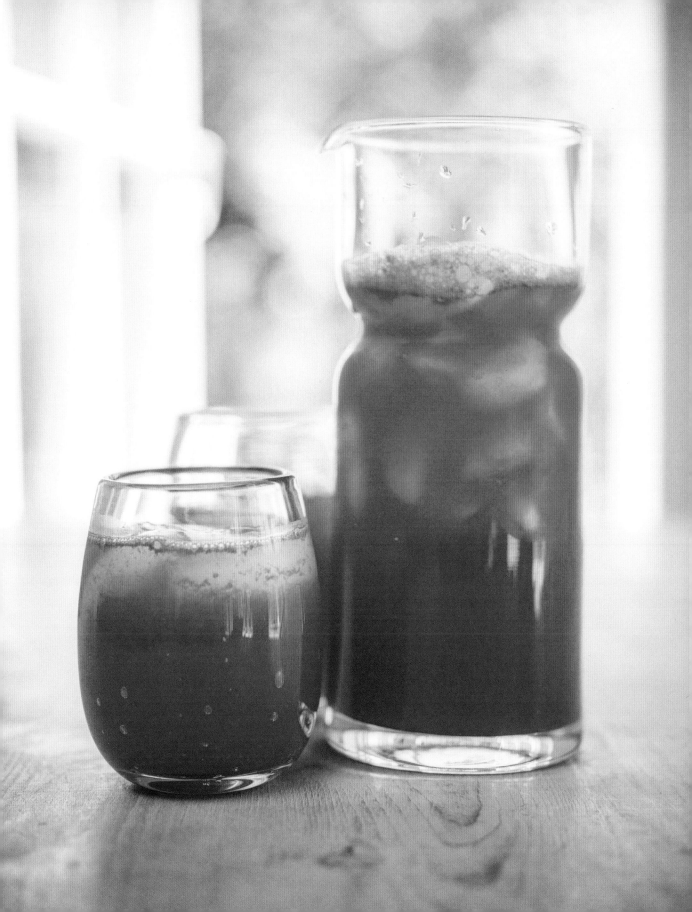

This is a simple but classic green juice. Kale is top of the green, leafy vegetables for flavour, antioxidants and vitamin content and it's now considered the go-to veg for green juices. I try to put it in everything I juice. I particularly love big old dinosaur kale leaves. If you struggle to get kale, though, substitute with spinach or chard.

ALL HAIL KALE

1 lemon, peeled

a handful of kale leaves

2 apples

2.5cm piece of fresh root ginger, peeled

Wash all your ingredients and peel where instructed. Juice them one by one in the order they are listed and serve chilled or enjoy over ice.

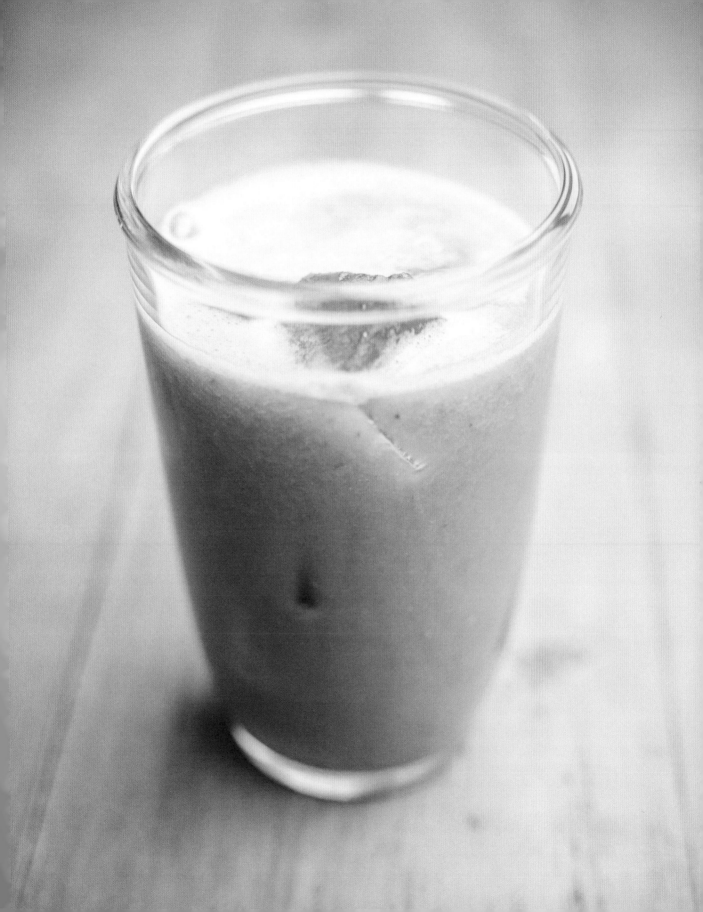

The benefits of beetroot juice are plenty – it was traditionally used to heal people. I like the taste, but beet juice can be a bit earthy. However, the oranges and ginger in this juice really balance out the flavour and make it super-delicious. Beets come in different shapes and colours, so try them all.

THE COLOUR OF RED

3 oranges, peeled

1cm piece of fresh root ginger, peeled

2 small beetroots (small to medium have the sweetest flavour), scrubbed

Wash all your ingredients and peel where instructed. Juice them one by one in the order they are listed and serve chilled or enjoy over ice.

JUICEMAN TIPS
This juice is great with the addition of pineapple. You can also add a teaspoon of wheatgrass powder to boost your energy.

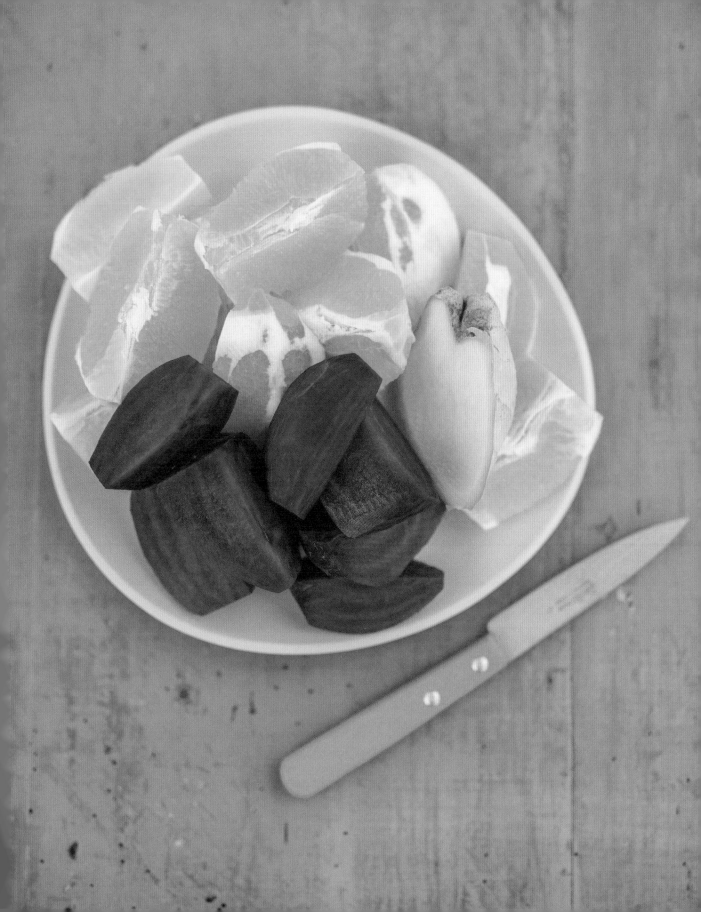

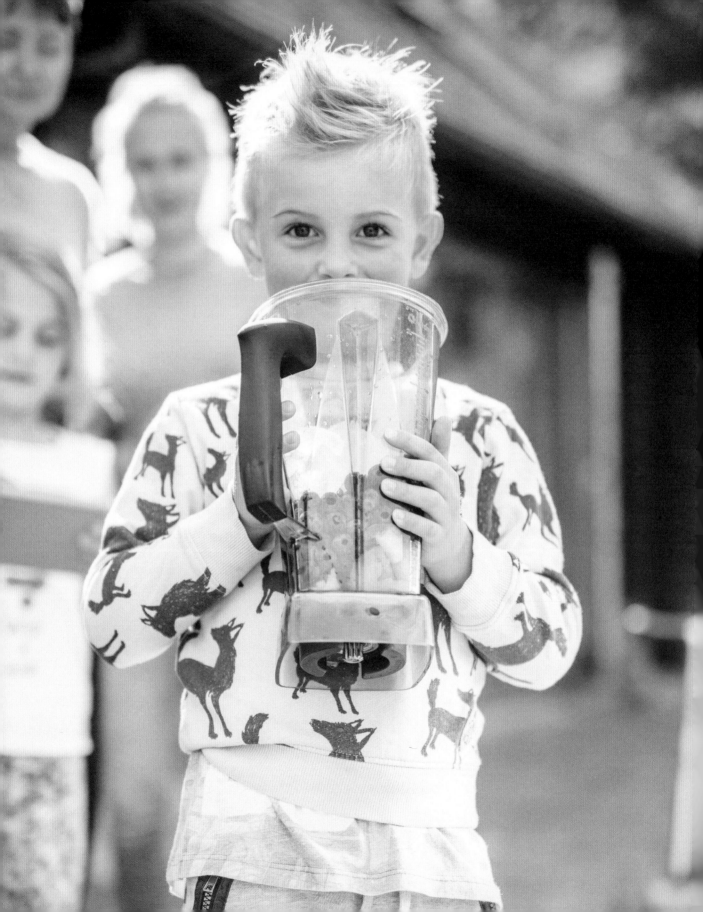

This is a great way to get your kids into new flavours. My little boy, Jackson, is mad for apple juice. I made him this juice one day when he was coming down with a cold to add some extra vits to his breakfast. He loves it, and so does his dad! I like to use Pink Lady apples and blood oranges if I can get organic ones.

JACKSON'S BREAKFAST JUICE

½ a lemon, peeled

1 kiwi fruit

1 orange, peeled

2 apples

Wash all your ingredients and peel where instructed. Juice them one by one in the order they are listed and serve chilled or enjoy over ice.

JUICEMAN TIPS
When peeling your orange, leave a thin layer of pith as it is a good source of vitamins. I like to leave the skin on the kiwis and simply chop them into chunks.

ORANGE HEALER

Apart from tasting delicious, this juice is full of immune-boosting vitamins. The black pepper helps to activate the curcumin in the turmeric and also adds a wonderful flavour.

1 orange, peeled

2.5cm piece of fresh root turmeric, peeled

½ a pineapple, peeled and cored

1 carrot

a pinch of black pepper

Wash all your ingredients and peel where instructed. Juice them one by one in the order they are listed, except for the black pepper. Serve chilled or enjoy over ice with the black pepper.

JUICEMAN TIPS
Add some ginger and a pinch of cinnamon for a touch of magic. Be careful when peeling turmeric as it can stain.

SKIN FOOD

Cucumber is naturally cooling, refreshing and super-hydrating, so it's brilliant for juicing. It also adds a lift to a jug of water for those warm summer days.

1 lime, peeled

a few mint leaves

¼ of a fennel bulb

½ a cucumber

½ an apple

Wash all your ingredients and peel the lime. Juice them one by one in the order they are listed, except for the mint. Serve chilled or enjoy over ice with the mint as a garnish.

JUICEMAN TIP
For extra power, add some chopped aloe vera leaf or a teaspoon of aloe vera juice.

DEEP GREEN

My mum brought me up on watercress soup, although the first time I cooked it myself I tried to blend the hot soup in a mixer and it spilled out everywhere and burned me! However, I wasn't put off and started introducing watercress into my juices. It does have a strong flavour, so you don't want to overdo it, but it's enjoyed a surge in popularity recently as one of the next big superfoods, so I try to include it where I can.

½ a lemon, peeled

a few sprigs of parsley

a handful of spinach leaves

a small handful of watercress

1 large kale leaf

2 celery sticks

¼ of a fennel bulb

½ a cucumber

Wash all your ingredients and peel where instructed. Juice them one by one in the order they are listed and serve chilled or enjoy over ice.

JUICEMAN TIP
For the hardcore juicers amongst you, add a teaspoon of spirulina or fresh wheatgrass for a superior boost.

COOL GREENS

Using fennel in your juice gives it a lovely flavour. It is slightly sweet and really refreshing. Fennel also contains high levels of minerals and vitamins, so it's a perfect addition to any juice.

½ a lemon, peeled

¼ of a fennel bulb

a handful of kale leaves

½ a large cucumber

2 apples

Wash all your ingredients and peel where instructed. Juice them one by one in the order they are listed and serve chilled or enjoy over ice.

JUICEMAN TIP
Mint is a great addition to this one.

This is a punchy, vibrant red juice with a massive vitamin content, and it's one of my favourite beet juices. I drink this before I go boxing. It's a great combo of sugars and spice to get you moving. A lot of famous sportsmen have said that they also drink beetroot juice before a workout, as it helps with energy and stamina.

This juice is packed with potassium, calcium and magnesium, topped with a good dose of vitamin C. The citrus from the grapefruit really balances the earthy beetroot. If you don't know what to do with your leftover fennel, try it dipped in hummus, or infused in warm water as a tummy tea.

BEET BOX

2.5cm piece of fresh
root ginger

½ a pink grapefruit, peeled

¼ of a fennel bulb

1 celery stick

1 beetroot, scrubbed

2 carrots

1 red apple

Wash all your ingredients and peel where instructed. Juice them one by one in the order they are listed and serve chilled or enjoy over ice.

JUICEMAN TIP
I tried this in New York with dandelion, which is a natural diuretic and very good for liver health. Get out in the fields if in season and add a leaf or two.

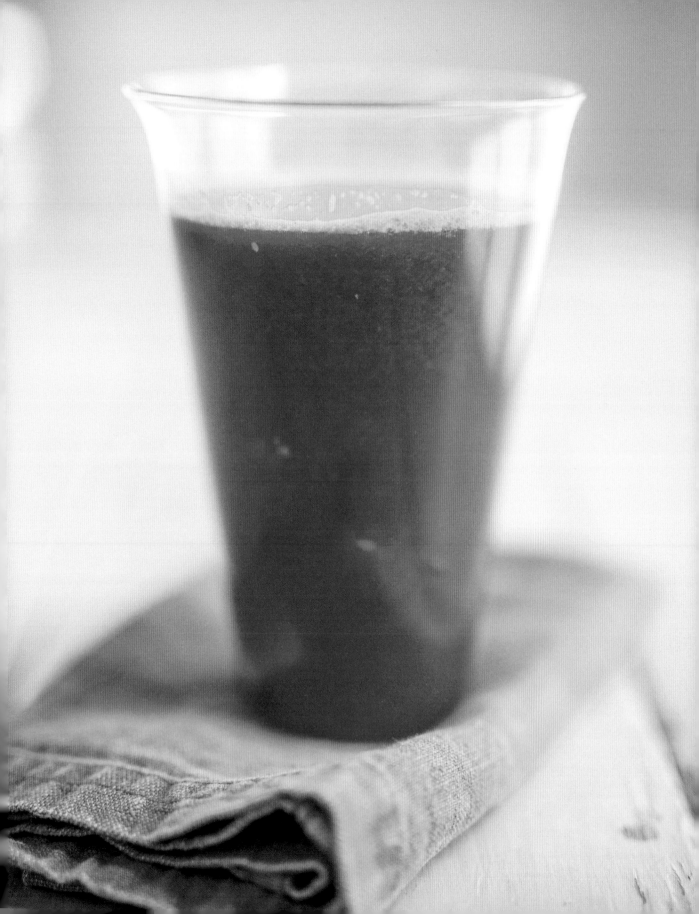

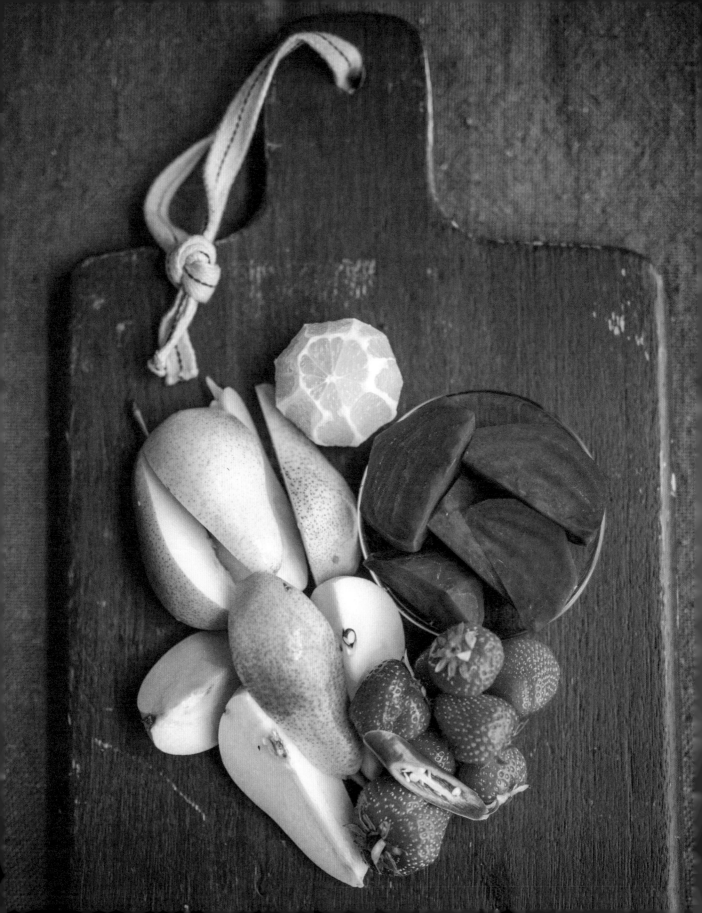

Sweet and spicy, this recipe has a gorgeous mix of ingredients. Don't underestimate the power of chilli (literally!) – it is packed with vitamin C, helps to boost metabolism and aids digestion. It also works really well with the lime, balancing the sweetness of the strawberries and pears.

HOT AND SWEET BEETS

a large handful
of strawberries

1 slice of red or green chilli

1 lime, peeled

1 beetroot, scrubbed

2 pears

Wash all your ingredients and peel where instructed. Juice them one by one in the order they are listed and serve chilled or enjoy over ice.

JUICEMAN TIP
If using organic strawberries, I like to leave the green tops on for added nutrients.

JUICEMAN FACT
Chillies and strawberries both have a higher vitamin C content than oranges.

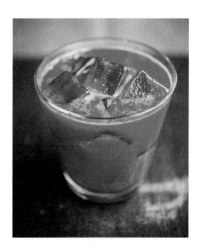

In the autumn months the UK has an abundance of pears. When we lived on a farm in Cheshire, I would juice pears every day for the kids. They're deliciously sweet and go great with ginger. This juice helps to soothe my stomach and digestion, while still tasting fantastic. It's a good one to have after lunch instead of dessert.

PINK HEALER

2.5cm piece of fresh
root ginger, peeled

½ a lime, peeled

1 tbsp aloe vera juice or
5cm aloe vera leaf, peeled

4 mint leaves

2 handfuls of strawberries

2 pears

Wash all your ingredients and peel where instructed. Juice them one by one in the order they are listed and serve chilled or enjoy over ice.

JUICEMAN TIPS
This juice makes great ice lollies. Leave out the ginger for a great family juice.

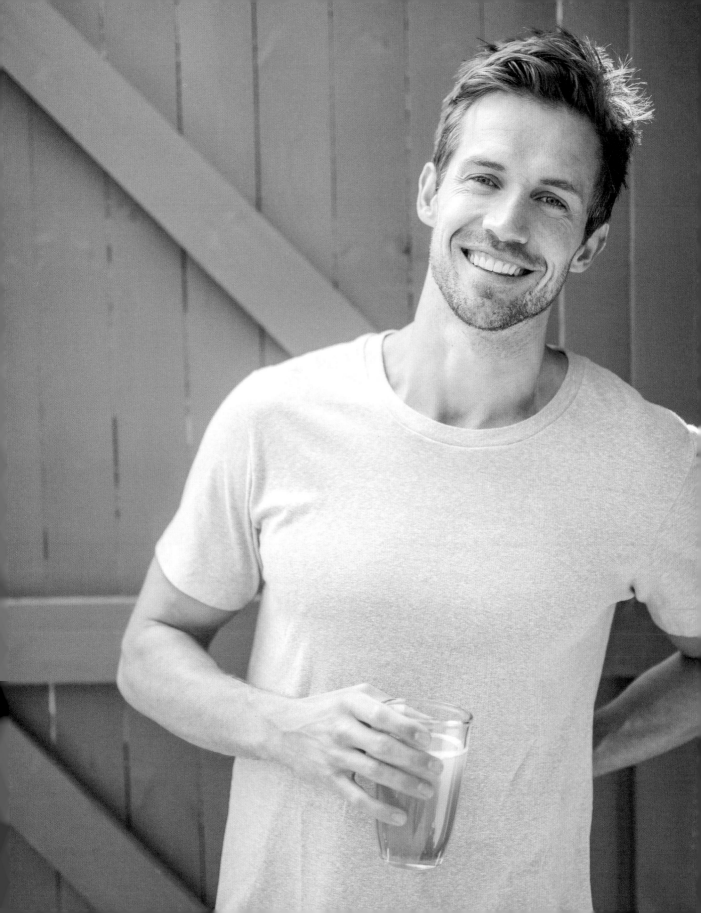

MEAN GREEN

This is an incredible juice packed with chlorophyll. I love coriander – it has quite a distinctive flavour and works especially well in a green juice. It has an unusual array of phytonutrients and antioxidants that makes it all the more beneficial.

2.5cm piece of fresh root ginger, peeled

½ a lime, peeled

a small bunch of coriander

a handful of kale leaves

2 celery sticks

1 pear

½ a large cucumber

Wash all your ingredients and peel where instructed. Juice them one by one in the order they are listed and serve chilled or enjoy over ice.

JUICEMAN TIP
I like to peel my ginger for a cleaner taste but the more earthy taste of unpeeled ginger can work well in some juices.

GREEN ROCKET

This is a serious energy-boosting juice and is loaded with goodness. It is a perfect low-sugar green juice. I like my juices green and this one is full of flavour from the lemongrass, coriander and ginger. You can play with the ginger levels on this one, but for me, the hotter the better.

2.5cm piece of fresh root ginger, peeled

1 lemon, peeled

½ a head of pak choi

a small bunch of coriander

2.5cm slice of lemongrass

1 chard leaf

1 kale leaf

1 celery stick

1 cucumber

Wash all your ingredients and peel where instructed. Juice them one by one in the order they are listed and serve chilled or enjoy over ice.

GREEN ROOTS

This is another perfect introduction to the world of green liquid, as there is a good balance of leafy greens, natural sugars and vitamin C. Carrot in a green juice works well and adds a light, sweet flavour. All my favourite vitamin-packed greens are in this one – providing a huge nutritional punch!

a small bunch of parsley

a handful of spinach leaves

1 kale leaf

2 carrots

1 celery stick

1 apple

½ a cucumber

Wash all your ingredients. Juice them one by one in the order they are listed and serve chilled or enjoy over ice.

JUICEMAN TIP
Add a sprinkle of ground cayenne pepper for some heat.

GREEN HERO

This juice is a great example of how creative you can be. Aloe vera is such a beneficial ingredient that I try to use it as much as possible. It is particularly good for cleansing the system. We have lots of aloe plants at home and they grow really well. When we are not using them in our juices, we are putting them on the kids' cuts and bruises to help them heal.

5cm piece of fresh root ginger, peeled

a handful of parsley

1 lemon, peeled

½ a pineapple, peeled and cored

1 cucumber

1 tbsp aloe vera juice
or 5cm aloe vera leaf, peeled

1 apple

1 tsp chia seeds

Wash all your ingredients, except the chia seeds, and peel where instructed. Juice them one by one in the order they are listed, then add the chia seeds and keep stirring until fully mixed. Serve chilled or enjoy over ice.

JUICEMAN TIP
Chia seeds swell in liquid, making them sticky, so stirring is important to ensure they don't clump together.

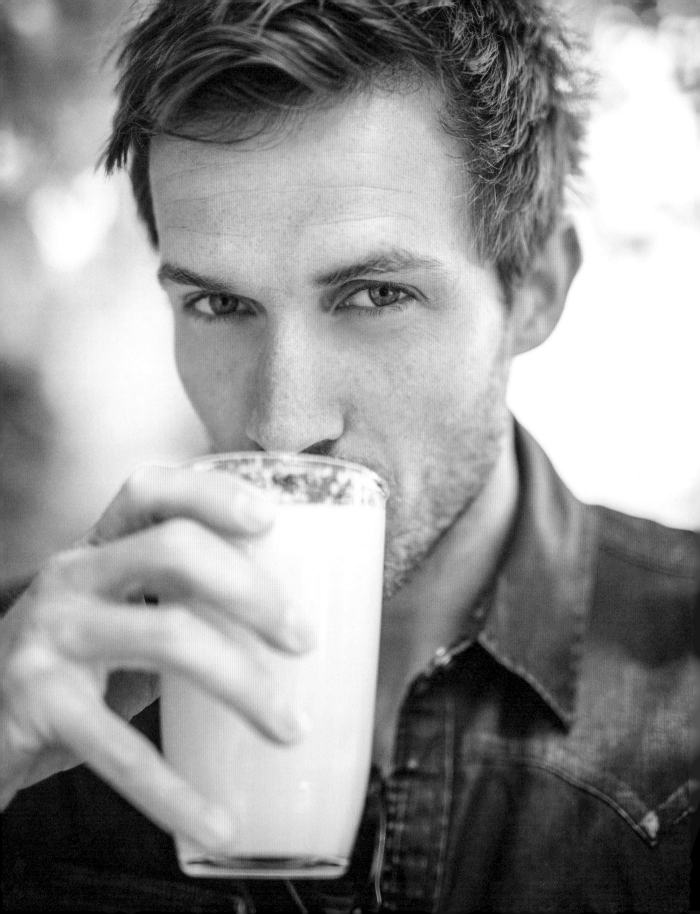

This is one of my favourite breakfast juices which I can drink bucketfuls of. I load it up with ginger – for me it's the more the better as it clears my head! It is quite addictive but full of vitamins, and great for aiding digestion. This is also one to keep in mind for cocktail night – I like to add a shot of tequila.

PPG

2.5cm piece of fresh
root ginger, peeled

½ a pineapple, peeled
and cored

2 pears, cored

Wash all your ingredients and peel where instructed. Juice them one by one in the order they are listed and serve chilled or enjoy over ice.

JUICEMAN FACT
Ginger is great for nausea. My wife was hooked on this juice when she was suffering from morning sickness.

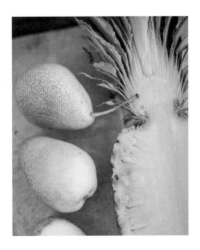

THE J5

Okay, this one is a Juiceman recipe and it's one of our bestsellers. It's a great juice for hydration and it tastes amazing. Chia seeds have a whole host of benefits: they contain protein and all the omegas and are a good source of energy. They work really well in a juice, as they expand in liquid and develop a gel-like texture.

¼ of a lemon, peeled	½ a cucumber
½ a pineapple, peeled and cored	1 tsp chia seeds

Wash all your ingredients, except the chia seeds, and peel where instructed. Juice them one by one in the order they are listed, and then add the chia seeds. Make sure you stir the chia seeds well so they do not stick together. Leave for 10 minutes or longer to allow the chia seeds to expand, then drink and enjoy.

JUICEMAN FACT
Gram for gram, chia seeds have 7.5 times more omega-3 than salmon.

SPICE IS NICE

This is one of my favourite juice recipes. Please don't be put off by the chilli in here – it works! Chillies also contain up to seven times more vitamin C than oranges and have a range of health benefits. I love spice but you can add less of the chilli and ginger – or more – to taste.

2.5cm piece of fresh root ginger, peeled	a small bunch of coriander
½ a lime, peeled	a handful of kale
1 thin slice of green chilli	3 apples

Wash all your ingredients and peel where instructed. Juice them one by one in the order they are listed and serve chilled or enjoy over ice.

JUICEMAN FACT
Chilli is great to kick-start your digestion and boost your metabolism.

GREEN NINJA

The fruit in this one makes it a super-yummy green juice. Put in as much spinach as you can for added nutrients. Blueberries are often talked about as a brain food, so don't underestimate the health benefits of the fruit here, too.

a handful of spinach leaves	2 apples
a handful of grapes	2 carrots
a handful of blueberries	½ a cucumber

Wash all your ingredients and juice them one by one in the order they are listed. Serve chilled or enjoy over ice.

JUICEMAN FACT
For a radiant glow, up your intake of blueberries as they're a powerful source of antioxidants. Grapes are very cleansing and the pips are full of essential fatty acids (grapeseed oils) that are amazing for skin and hair.

COOL AS A CUCUMBER

Cucumbers are perfect for juicing, as they are 96 per cent water, making them great for hydration while still having a high vitamin content. I would definitely recommend buying organic cucumbers, as they are ranked the twelfth most contaminated food. However, the good news is that finding organic cucumbers in the supermarket is really easy these days.

1 lime, peeled	2 celery sticks
a small handful of mint	1 cucumber

Wash all your ingredients and peel where instructed. Juice them one by one in the order they are listed and serve chilled or enjoy over ice.

JUICEMAN TIP
This juice makes great ice cubes – perfect to put in a jug of water.

JUICEMAN FACT
Cucumbers grow really well in the UK and are a firm favourite in allotments.

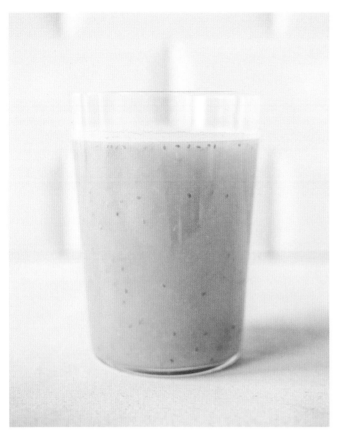

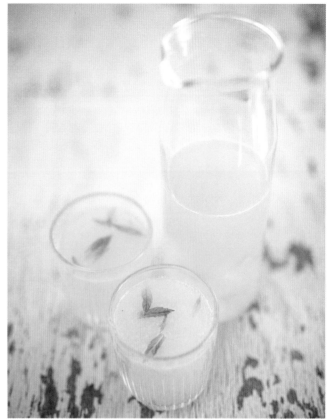

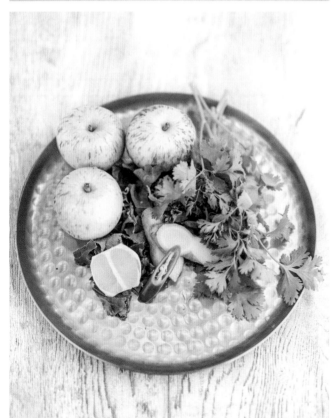

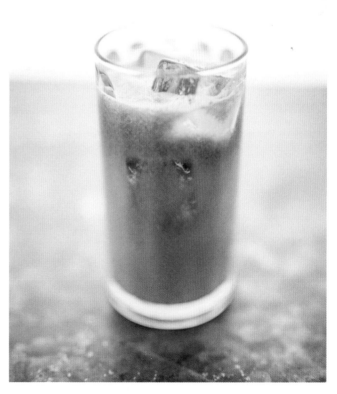

This juice is a summer classic. I designed it for my daughter, Taylor, to give her an energy boost before she played tennis. It's a firm favourite with her friends too – including Stella in the picture. I make it for them using the lime, and I have it with the ginger. It looks and tastes great, and we make the most of the organic strawberries available in the summer months.

WIMBLEDON WINNER

2.5cm piece of fresh root ginger, peeled, or 1 lime, peeled

2 handfuls of strawberries

½ a pineapple, peeled and cored

1 small beetroot, scrubbed

Wash all your ingredients and peel where instructed. Juice them one by one in the order they are listed and serve chilled or enjoy over ice.

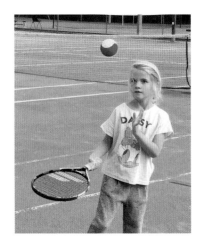

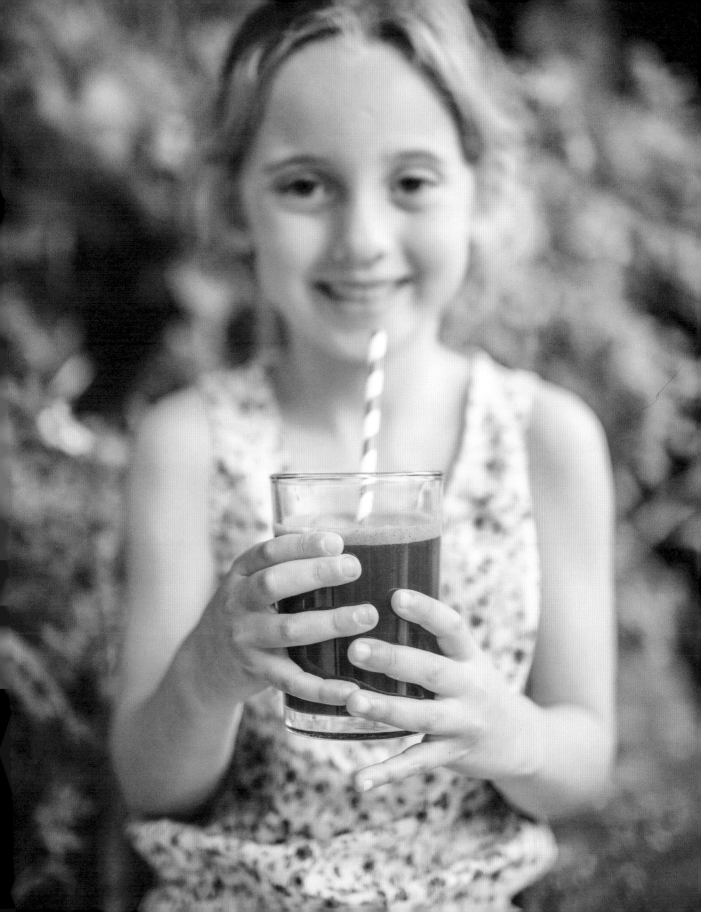

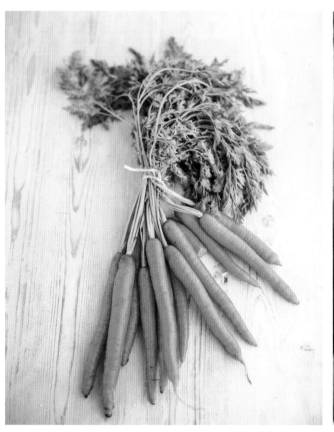
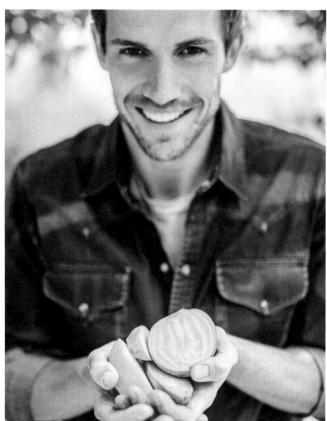
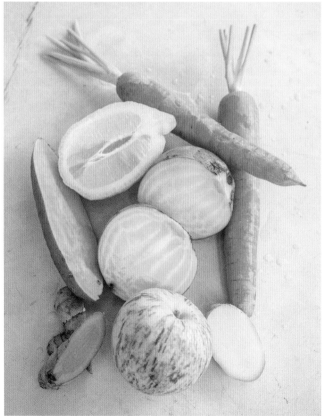
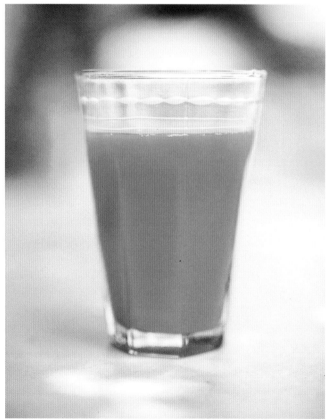

This juice is spectacular – you must try it. I am a huge fan of carrots and sweet potato, as they are renowned for their amazing health benefits. The curcumin in turmeric is stronger than vitamin C and five to eight times stronger than vitamin E in terms of its immunity-boosting abilities. When I drink this juice I feel great.

ULTIMATE OJ

2.5cm piece of fresh root turmeric, peeled

½ a lemon, peeled

2.5cm piece of fresh root ginger, peeled

1 yellow beetroot, scrubbed

½ a sweet potato, scrubbed

2 carrots

1 apple

Wash all your ingredients and peel where instructed. Juice them one by one in the order they are listed and serve chilled or enjoy over ice.

JUICEMAN FACT
Turmeric is the mother of anti-inflammatory foods. If you can't find fresh turmeric, stir in a teaspoon of ground.

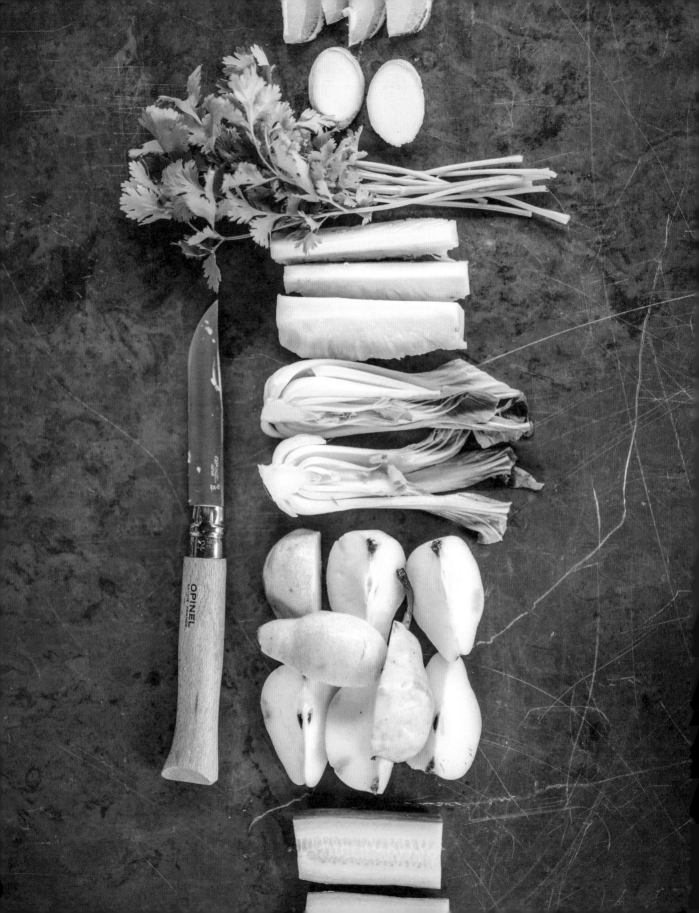

Let's be straight: if it grows and it's green, it can be juiced – even pak choi. Not only is it full of vitamin C, vitamin K, calcium and antioxidants, it also has a subtle taste, making it perfect for first-time juicers. I remember drinking the best pineapple juice in Koh Samui and eating an amazing green curry, which together inspired this recipe.

THAI GREEN

2.5cm piece of fresh
root ginger, peeled

1 lime, peeled

a handful of coriander

1 head of pak choi

¼ of a pineapple, peeled
and cored

2 pears

¼ of a cucumber

Wash all your ingredients and peel where instructed. Juice them one by one in the order they are listed and serve chilled or enjoy over ice.

JUICEMAN TIP
Add a slice of lemongrass and a slice of chilli for extra Thai vibes.

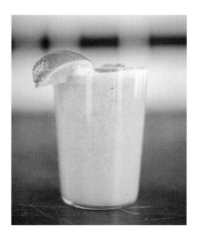

This is a great example of a really tasty fruit juice that's both hydrating and nourishing. Melons are such a great ingredient, as they are hydrating, energy-boosting and super-low in calories all at the same time. The ginger kick will boost your metabolism, making this a perfect pre-workout drink.

SKINNY JEANS

2.5cm piece of fresh root ginger, peeled

½ a medium-sized cantaloupe melon, peeled

1 slice of watermelon, peeled

3 carrots

Wash all your ingredients and peel where instructed. Juice them one by one in the order they are listed and serve chilled or enjoy over ice.

JUICEMAN TIP
I often add a 2.5cm piece of fresh root turmeric to this recipe.

JUICEMAN FACT
You can also juice the rind of a melon. It's not as sweet as the flesh but it contains a number of nutrients.

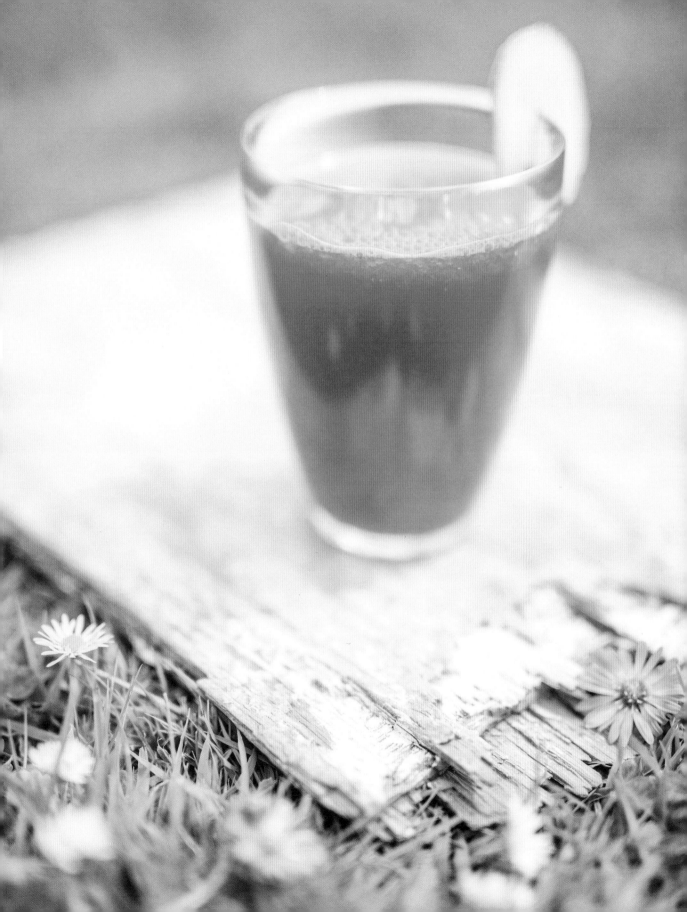

Sweet and spicy is my thing. This juice was first created at Juiceman HQ when we were sent a palette of raspberries that were about to go off. We put this juice together and it was an instant success. Organic raspberries are easy to find at the supermarket nowadays, so this can be a regular treat. The lemon and chilli prevent it from being too sweet and the result is utterly delicious.

RASPBERRY KICKER

¼ of a lemon, peeled

1 slice of red chilli

2 handfuls of raspberries

3 apples

Wash all your ingredients and peel where instructed. Juice them one by one in the order they are listed and serve chilled or enjoy over ice.

JUICEMAN TIPS
Try freezing some raspberries to serve on top with a sprig of mint. Add a shot of rum to turn this juice into a delicious cocktail.

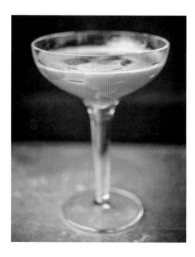

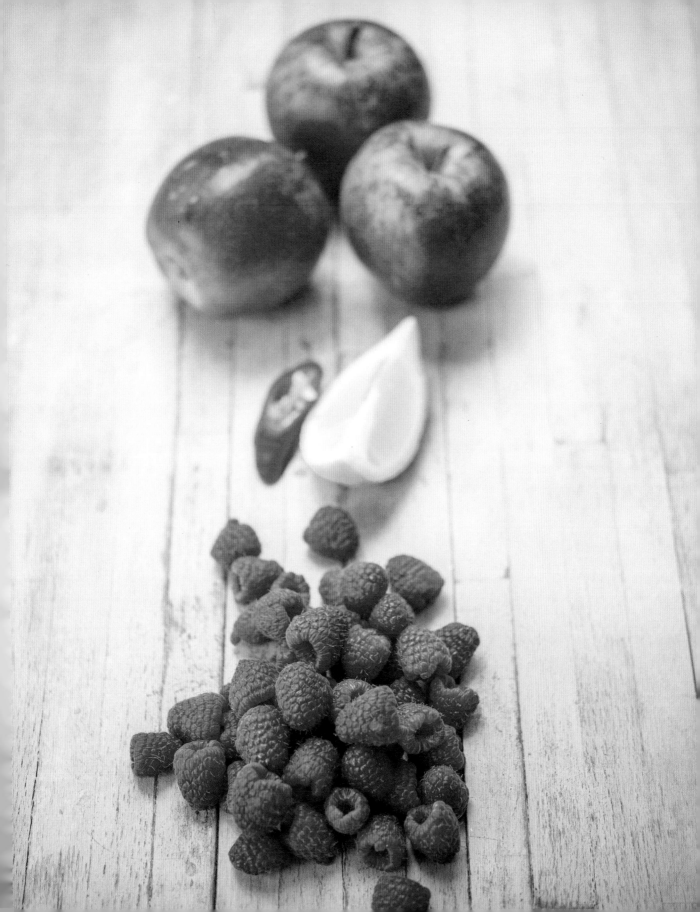

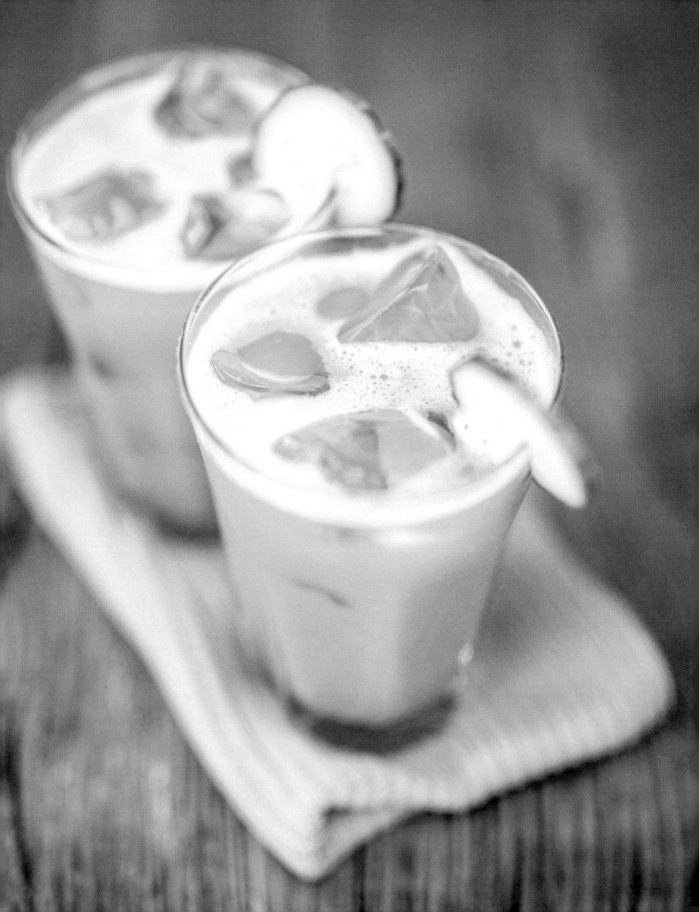

Don't be put off by the idea of drinking your salad. Romaine lettuce is a great addition to a green juice. This is my wife's favourite juice – she says it makes her skin glow. Parsley is an amazing herb to add to your juices. It is super-rich in chlorophyll, which is the energy-producing substance that gives herbs and plants their characteristic green colour.

GREEN GLOW

2.5cm piece of fresh root ginger, peeled

1 lemon, peeled

a small handful of flat-leaf parsley

a handful of spinach leaves

½ a romaine lettuce, outer leaves removed

1 pear

1 large or 2 small cucumbers

Wash all your ingredients and peel where instructed. Juice them one by one in the order they are listed and serve chilled or enjoy over ice.

JUICEMAN FACT
Romaine lettuce is supercharged with vitamin K, great for bone health.

I find that using pineapple in a green juice makes it taste super-good, and this is one of my favourite examples. This juice also uses courgettes, which have a subtle flavour and are perfect for juices. When I had my own allotment, courgettes were so easy to grow that I juiced them regularly.

GREEN LOVE

¼ of a lemon, peeled

2.5cm piece of fresh root ginger, peeled

½ a courgette

¼ of a fennel bulb

¼ of a pineapple, peeled and cored

1 celery stick

1 pear

Wash all your ingredients and peel where instructed. Juice them one by one in the order they are listed and serve chilled or enjoy over ice.

JUICEMAN TIP
If you like turning your courgettes into courgetti, these ingredients also make a great summer salad.

JUICEMAN FACT
The darker varieties of courgettes have more nutrients.

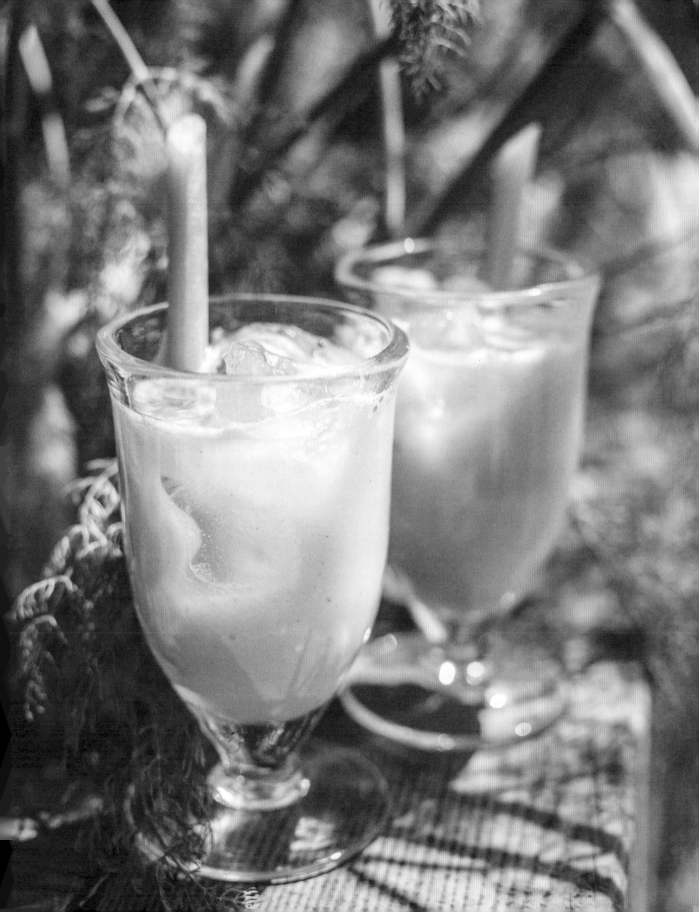

This is a classic way of taking full advantage of what's in season. I was run-down one winter and feeling a cold coming on. As we had an abundance of rhubarb, I chucked a load in to my juices and loved it. This is now my go-to recipe for when I need to give my immune system a boost and fight off a cold. It also tastes surprisingly good. Rosemary is a great herb to help open the airways, as it's aromatic.

WINTER COLD KICKER

5cm piece of fresh root ginger, peeled

2.5cm piece of fresh root turmeric, peeled

a few leaves of fresh rosemary

1 lemon, peeled

1 orange, peeled

a handful of grapes

1 rhubarb stick (if in season)

3 celery sticks

8 drops of echinacea extract

a pinch of cayenne pepper

Wash all your ingredients, except the echinacea extract and cayenne pepper, and peel where instructed. Juice them one by one in the order they are listed, then add the echinacea and cayenne to taste, stir and enjoy over ice.

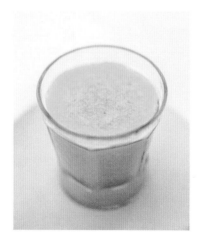

This is a powerful green juice. Chard, although
a green, leafy vegetable, is actually a member
of the beet family – so it tastes a bit like spinach
and a bit like beetroot. It is a nutritional powerhouse,
so if you see it, buy it and juice it!

LOVE IT SPICY GREEN

2.5cm piece of fresh root
ginger, peeled

1 lemon, peeled

½ a bunch of watercress

a handful of mixed chard
and kale leaves

½ a romaine lettuce

2 celery sticks

2 small apples

a pinch of ground cayenne
pepper

Wash all your ingredients, except the cayenne
pepper, and peel where instructed. Juice them
one by one in the order they are listed, then
add the cayenne pepper to taste. Stir and
serve chilled or enjoy over ice.

JUICEMAN TIP
Any kale or chard left over will work brilliantly
in a salad when raw.

JUICEMAN FACT
Kale juice contains more calcium than
a glass of milk.

This juice does what it says on the label. The ingredients will help alkalise your pH level. Much has been said about the benefits of an alkaline diet and I personally agree that it will help to maintain health and keep illness at bay.

ALKALISE

½ a lemon, peeled

a small bunch of flat-leaf parsley

2 handfuls of mixed greens (kale, spinach and chard)

3 celery sticks

1 apple

Wash all your ingredients and peel where instructed. Juice them one by one in the order they are listed and serve chilled or enjoy over ice.

JUICEMAN TIP
Magnesium is known to help induce sleep and, as celery is high in magnesium, this is a great juice to have in the evening.

JUICEMAN FACT
Celery is packed with phenolic antioxidants, which have been shown to provide many anti-inflammatory benefits.

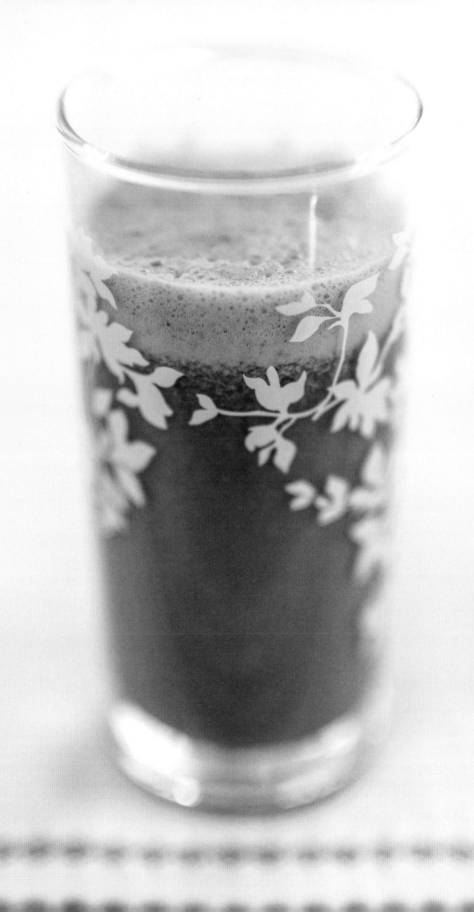

Sometimes it's nice to add water to a juice to create a tonic. This is more of a tonic than a juice. It's gorgeously refreshing and great to serve when you have friends over, especially during barbecue season.

PINEAPPLEADE

1 lemon, peeled

½ a pineapple, peeled and cored

1 tbsp agave syrup

750ml mineral water

Wash your ingredients, except the agave syrup, and peel where instructed. Juice the lemon and pineapple, then pour into a jug with the agave and mineral water, stir and leave in the fridge. You can save some pineapple chunks and slices of ginger to serve with it.

JUICEMAN TIP
This recipe also works really well with ginger for added heat.

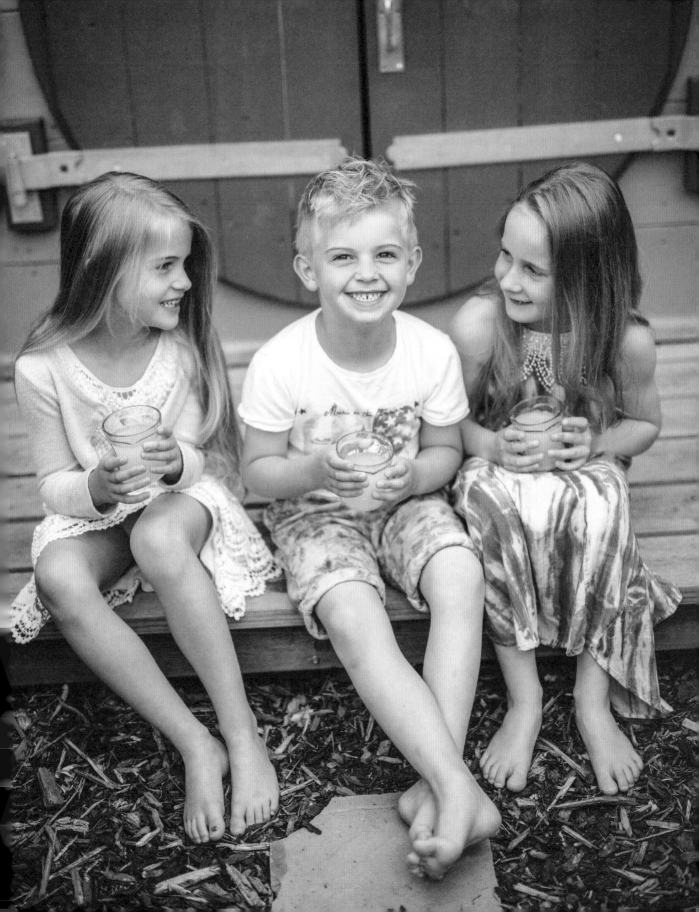

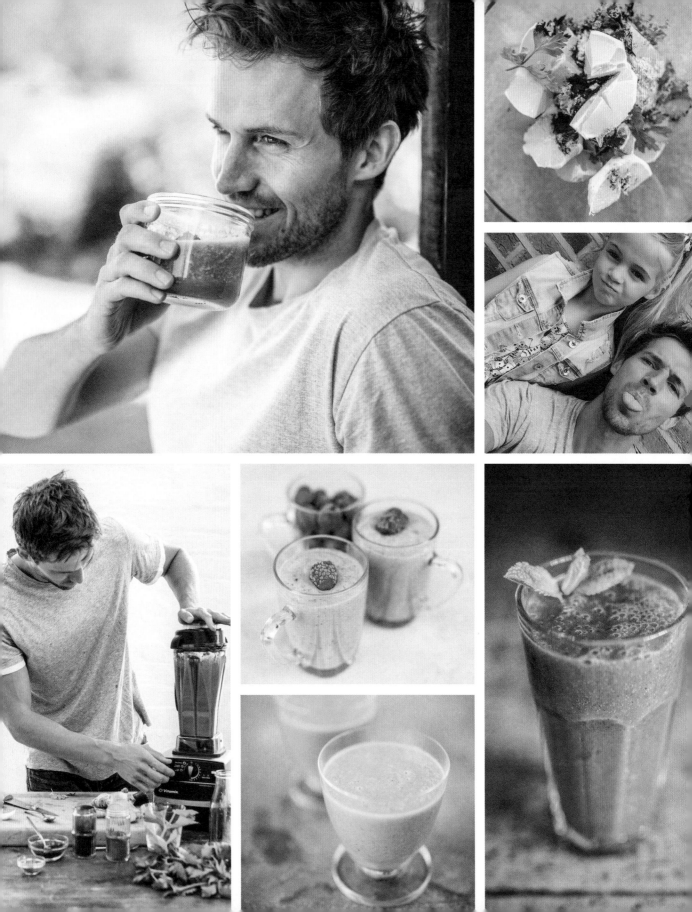

SMOOTHIES

The main difference between a smoothie and a juice is the fibre content. The fibre is removed from juices making the liquid much thinner. So if you want something more substantial, a smoothie is for you. There is also no pulp waste with a smoothie as the whole ingredient is used.

I just love smoothies. I find that they're a brilliant way to start the day or have a meal when I don't have time to cook. They provide all the raw goodness of a juice plus fibre and enzymes. Whether you are into all-green super smoothies or nut milkshakes, you can always tailor the recipe with some hidden supplements depending on the time of day, your physical state or simply how you're feeling. For example, if you need some energy you can add extra dates, cacao powder or a shot of espresso to a nut milk, or if you're in need of some recovery, it's as simple as throwing in a scoop of hemp protein and some chia seeds.

One of the best things about smoothies is that you can hide the stuff you usually don't like but know is good for you. For example, my little man Jackson is not fond of spinach and would never eat a handful of raw spinach. But in a smoothie it's all good.

The recipes in this chapter make 1 large glass or 2 smaller glasses.

Embrace your blender and keep it out and in constant use all day: from a smoothie bowl for breakfast or a protein shake after yoga, to making hummus or guacamole in the evening.

Here are some great techniques to get the best out of your shopping and blender. Simple things like making smoothie bags of ripe fruit for specific recipes will go a long way towards making sure you get the best out of this section.

FROZEN FRUIT

One of the biggest problems with juicing and making smoothies is the fact that you want to use fresh ingredients that are ripe but not too ripe. The answer is to buy fruit and veg when in season and once perfectly ripe, freeze them. The best bags for this are ziplock freezer bags. I always buy soft fruits like strawberries and bananas in bulk and freeze them.

HOW TO BULK FREEZE YOUR FRUIT:

Banana: when ripe, peel and cut into cubes to freeze

Pineapple: peel the skin, cut into chunks and then freeze

Blueberries, raspberries and strawberries: very seasonal, so when you see some organic ones, buy them, wash them and freeze. You can freeze the strawberries with the green on the top. I never actually bother cutting these off.

Melon: peel, scoop out the pips, cut into chunks and freeze

Apples and pears: wash, core, cut into chunks and freeze

This is such a great way to get ahead of yourself. I would recommend storing for a maximum of 6 months.

KEEP YOUR BLENDER HAPPY

Here are a few tips for keeping a happy blender:

- Don't overfill unless you wanna wear it. Make sure the lid is on before starting it up.

- Soak all nuts and seeds to keep a happy blender engine.

- Chop and grate where possible, depending on your model. It's important not to overheat your smoothies, which will make them warm . . . Yuck!

- Put ingredients in the blender in the right order:

  Liquid
  Powders
  Solids
  Ice and frozen stuff

- Blend initially at a quarter power for 20 seconds and then gradually increase to full power. Blitz for 30 seconds until smooth. Just add more liquid for a runnier consistency.

- Clean immediately after every use with warm soapy water. If you leave it then you will have a hard time later.

This smoothie has lots of ingredients that are great for your skin. I love melons, as they are one of the best natural sources of antioxidants and contain vitamins A and C – all of which help your body fight off the signs of ageing.

SKIN LOVE

250ml mineral water

½ a grapefruit, peeled and chopped

¼ of a cantaloupe melon, peeled and chopped

a small handful of basil

2 Medjool dates, pitted

2 cucumbers, chopped

Wash, peel and chop the ingredients where necessary. Put all the ingredients into a blender in the order they're listed. Blitz until smooth.

JUICEMAN TIP
The basil can be substituted for coriander or parsley. I also like to add some ginger for added zing.

JUICEMAN FACT
Cucumbers are 96 per cent water and very hydrating.

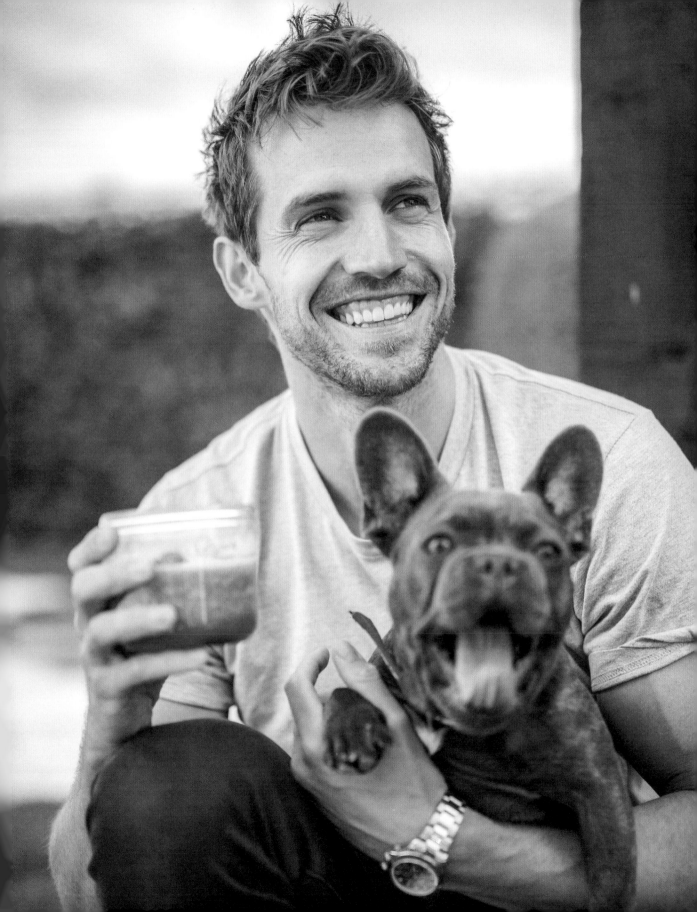

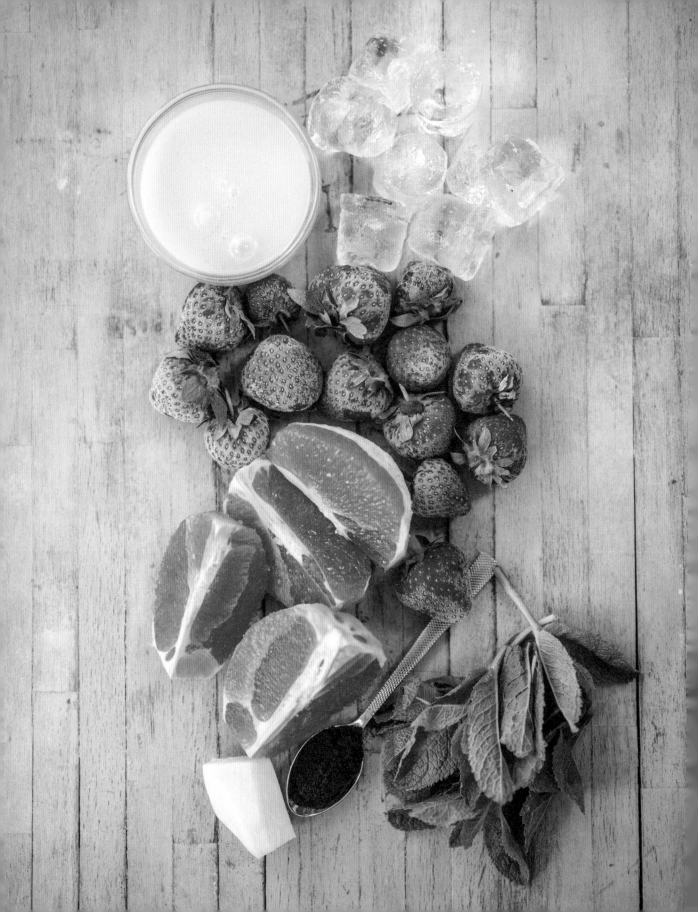

I find that whenever I'm feeling run-down I look for ways to incorporate extra vitamin C into my diet. Grapefruits are a brilliant source and taste delicious with sweeter ingredients such as strawberries. This is a great pick-me-up smoothie. It's like a punchy strawberry milkshake. As it's packed with vitamin C, it will give you energy and an immunity boost when you need it.

IMMUNITY BOOST

300ml coconut or almond milk

1½ tsp vanilla powder

a small bunch of mint

2.5cm piece of fresh root ginger, peeled

1 red grapefruit, peeled and chopped

2 handfuls of frozen strawberries

a handful of ice cubes

Wash, peel and chop the ingredients where necessary. Put all the ingredients into a blender in the order they're listed. Blitz until smooth.

JUICEMAN TIP
Sprinkle with hemp seeds and chia seeds for added protein and omegas.

JUICEMAN FACT
Vanilla is a great antioxidant.

If I need to get fired up in the morning, this is the smoothie that does the job. The chilli gives a kick of flavour as well as a boost to your metabolism. The recipe also contains two of my favourite superfoods: flaxseeds and hemp seeds. Hemp is a complete source of protein, and the oil from the seeds has one of the highest percentages of essential fatty acids of any seed. Flaxseeds are a great source of fibre, protein and omega-3, all of which help your cardiovascular system.

FIRE-STARTER

350ml almond milk

1 tbsp flaxseeds

3 tbsp hemp seeds

1cm slice of red chilli

½ a lime, peeled

a handful of chopped mango

a handful of frozen raspberries

½ a frozen banana

Wash, peel and chop the ingredients where necessary. Put all the ingredients into a blender in the order they're listed. Blitz until smooth.

JUICEMAN TIP
Keep a good supply of raspberries in the freezer for when they're not in season. They're really easy to grow too.

JUICEMAN FACT
Almond milk is a great source of vitamin E.

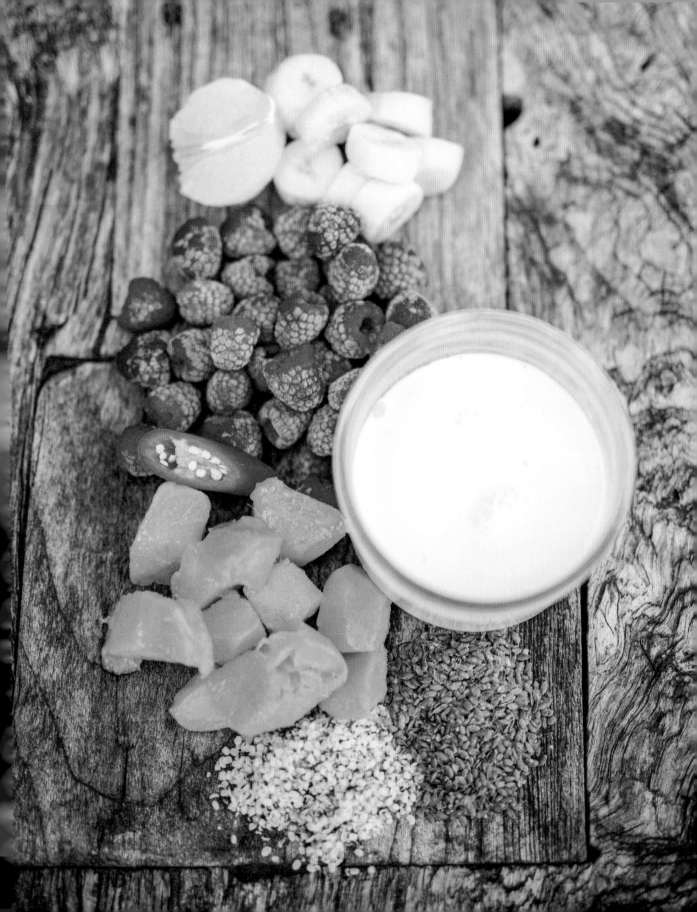

This smoothie is so good – it is hydrating and superpowered. I like to drink this when I come out of the gym. It has everything I need to help my body recover after a workout and replenish its energy levels. Recovery from exercise is vital for keeping up your immunity and staying well. This recipe also makes a great meal replacement.

RECOVERY SHAKE

325ml coconut water, or coconut or almond milk

1 tbsp natural protein powder

1 tsp greens powder or spirulina

1 tsp chia seeds

1 tbsp goji berries

¼ of a romaine lettuce

¼ of an avocado, peeled and destoned

¼ of a pineapple, peeled and cored

3 handfuls of frozen blueberries

Wash, peel and chop the ingredients where necessary. Put all the ingredients into a blender in the order they're listed. Blitz until smooth.

JUICEMAN FACT
Spirulina is one of the leading sources of GLA (gamma-linolenic acid), which is one of the most powerful anti-inflammatory agents in nature. GLA is also particularly beneficial to women, as it can ease pre-menstrual symptoms. Gram for gram, spirulina also contains 26 times the calcium of milk.

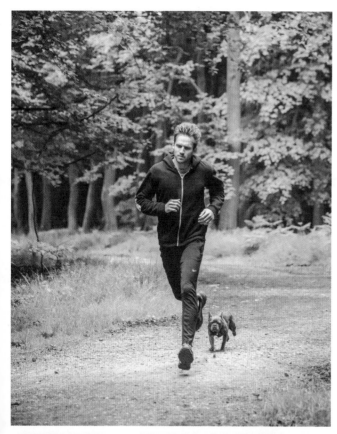

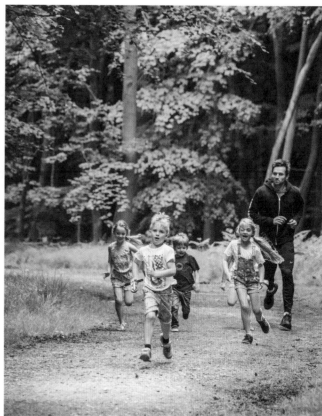

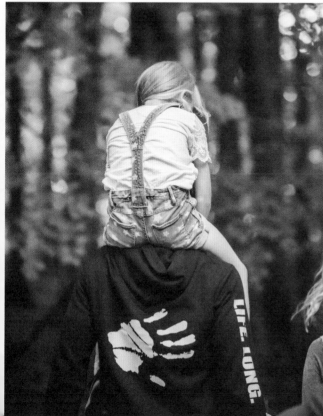

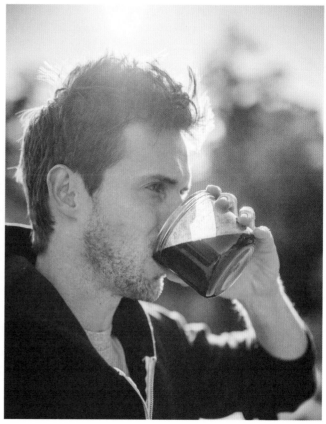

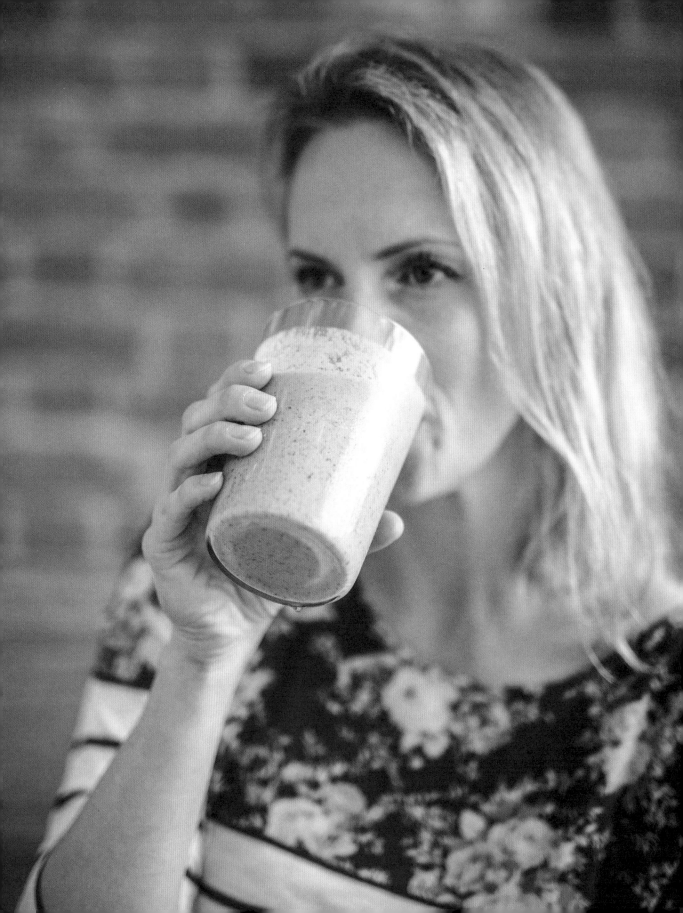

This smoothie, in my mind, is the key to my very healthy son, Jackson. I was obsessing over smoothies during Jane's pregnancy and we would have one every day that was high in folic acid and iron from the spinach and the kale. It's true that you are what you eat, and this certainly seems to be the case for my strong son. He hit the ground running and was necking green smoothies with his dad from six months old, and I swear he is very rarely ill and a happy little chap. This recipe makes a great breakfast smoothie. It's also a definite power snack and is probably one of my favourites.

SUPERMUM

400ml almond milk or milk of your choice

1 tbsp hemp oil

1 tsp wheatgrass powder

1 tbsp flaxseeds

a pinch of vanilla powder

a few mint leaves

a handful of spinach leaves (fresh or frozen)

a few kale leaves

¼ of a cucumber, chopped

2 Medjool dates, pitted

½ an avocado, peeled and destoned

a handful of frozen strawberries

1 frozen banana

Wash, peel and chop the ingredients where necessary. Put all the ingredients into a blender in the order they're listed. Blitz until smooth.

JUICEMAN FACTS
Healthy oils are incredibly important. Hemp oil is easily digested and contains all the necessary essential amino acids and essential fatty acids. It's also great if you're feeling fatigued.

My daughter makes this one with me. We have added extra ingredients since we first started making it, and I have explained to her what they are and why they are so good for us. It started off with just blueberries, raspberries and oranges! It's a great smoothie to add some secret veggies to. A handful of spinach works a treat.

TAYLOR'S FAVOURITE TIPPLE

350ml coconut
or almond milk

1 tsp ground cinnamon

½ tsp vanilla powder

1 tsp hemp oil

2 oranges, peeled

1 kiwi fruit

2 handfuls of frozen
raspberries

2 handfuls of frozen
blueberries

Wash, peel and chop the ingredients where necessary. Put all the ingredients into a blender in the order they're listed. Blitz until smooth.

JUICEMAN TIP
Throw in a teaspoon of spirulina for an extra health kick.

JUICEMAN FACT
Kiwis are packed with vitamins C and K, great for keeping your immune system strong.

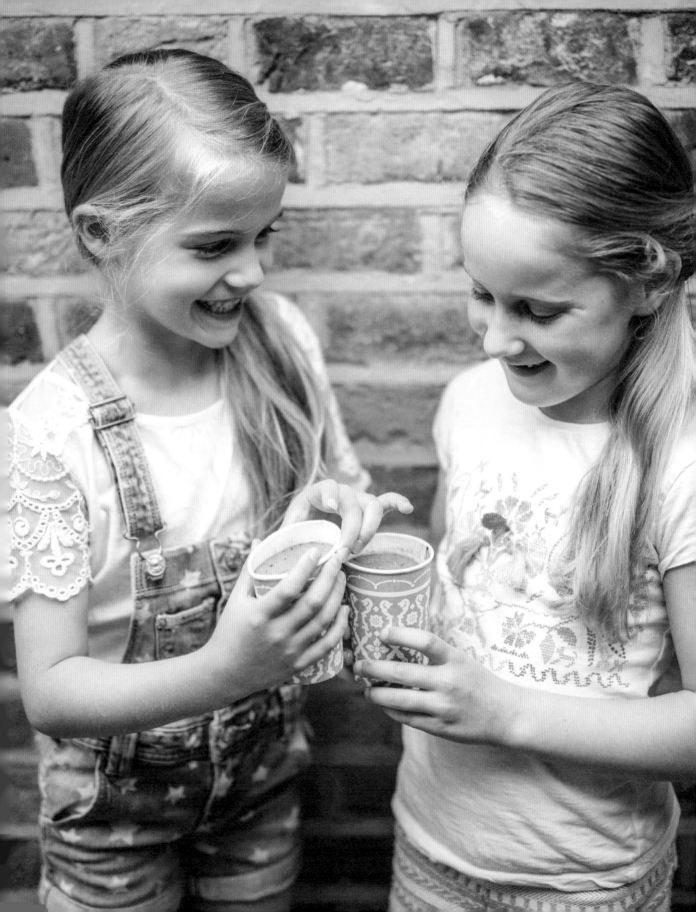

BLUEBERRY FACIAL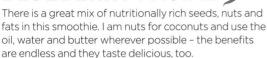

There is a great mix of nutritionally rich seeds, nuts and fats in this smoothie. I am nuts for coconuts and use the oil, water and butter wherever possible – the benefits are endless and they taste delicious, too.

300ml coconut water	2 tbsp coconut flakes or coconut butter
2.5cm piece of fresh root ginger, peeled and chopped	a small handful of pumpkin seeds
1 lime, peeled	1 frozen banana
a handful of walnuts	2 handfuls of frozen blueberries

Wash, peel and chop the ingredients where necessary. Put all the ingredients into a blender in the order they're listed. Blitz until smooth.

JUICEMAN TIP
Coconut oil makes an amazing body moisturiser.

JUICEMAN FACT
Walnuts are full of omega-3 and are a beauty food.

THE INCREDIBLES

My kids love this one. It's yummy, creamy and sweet, just like a milkshake. They have no idea that it's good for them!

2 handfuls of spinach leaves	a pinch of ground cinnamon
½ an avocado, peeled and destoned	2 Medjool dates, pitted
350ml liquid of your choice (coconut milk, almond milk or coconut water)	1 tsp raw honey
	2 frozen bananas

Wash, peel and chop the ingredients where necessary. Put all the ingredients into a blender in the order they're listed. Blitz until smooth.

JUICEMAN TIP
Add a tablespoon of chia seeds and half a teaspoon of spirulina to superpower this smoothie.

LOVE PURPLE

This is a smoothie for the entire family. The mix of fruit and yogurt gives it a high yummy rating. Dates are a great addition to any smoothie – they don't just add sweetness, they are also a good source of fibre, which is essential for a healthy and efficient digestive system. This one is also great served with chopped fruit and granola for breakfast.

100–200g Greek yogurt or coconut yogurt	1 plum, pitted and chopped
a handful of ice cubes	1 peach, pitted and chopped
a few mint leaves	3 handfuls of frozen blueberries
1 Medjool date, pitted	150ml coconut water

Wash, peel and chop the ingredients where necessary. Put all the ingredients into a blender in the order they're listed. Blitz until smooth.

STRAWBERRY MILKSHAKE

This smoothie is a great energy-boosting way to start the day. Organic strawberries are hard to find all year round, so to enjoy this healthy milkshake at any time of year keep lots of them in the freezer. Feel free to add a date or two for extra fibre and sweetness. Top with hemp seeds, pumpkin seeds and bee pollen.

1 frozen banana	1 tbsp nut butter
½ an avocado, peeled and destoned	2 handfuls of strawberries (fresh or frozen)
½ a lime, peeled	a pinch of vanilla powder
325ml almond or other nut milk, or milk of your choice	

Wash, peel and chop the ingredients where necessary. Put all the ingredients into a blender in the order they're listed. Blitz until smooth.

JUICEMAN TIPS
This makes a great protein shake by adding a tablespoon of protein powder of your choice (see p.16). You can turn this into a chocolate milkshake by substituting the strawberries for a tablespoon of cacao powder, or a banana milkshake by adding an extra banana (fresh or frozen) instead of the strawberries.

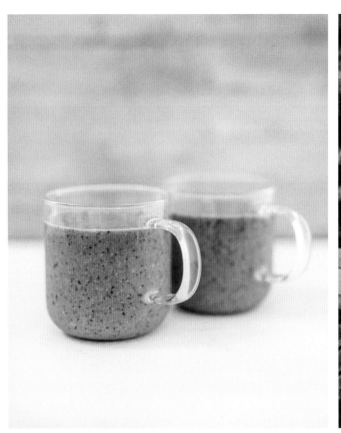

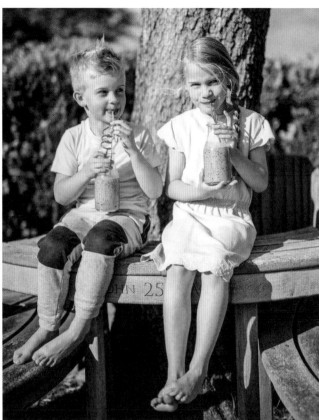

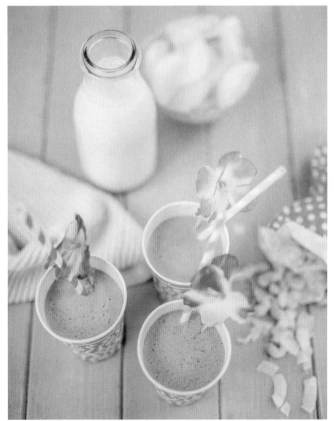

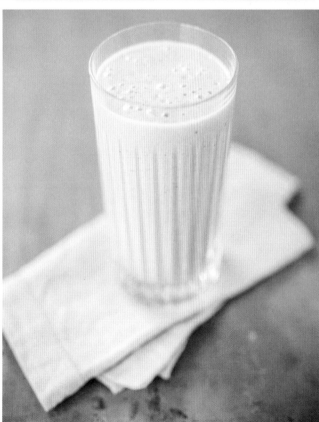

I love this bad boy after a workout. Anyone who likes chocolate: cacao is your friend. It is raw chocolate and contains more than 300 nutritional compounds. It's also one of the richest sources of antioxidants of any food on the planet. Chocolate-flavoured protein powder works really well here.

CHOCOLATE REBEL

350ml mineral water

a pinch of Himalayan salt

1 tbsp natural protein powder

1 tsp coconut oil

1 tbsp raw honey or maple syrup

1 tbsp hemp seeds

5 cashew nuts

3 tbsp raw cacao powder

1 tbsp raw cacao nibs

½ an avocado

1 frozen banana

a handful of frozen strawberries

a handful of ice cubes

Wash, peel and chop the ingredients where necessary. Put all the ingredients into a blender in the order they're listed. Blitz until smooth.

JUICEMAN TIP
Add maca powder for an added energy boost and top with goji berries, hemp seeds and cacao nibs.

JUICEMAN FACT
Cacao has 10 times more antioxidants than green tea.

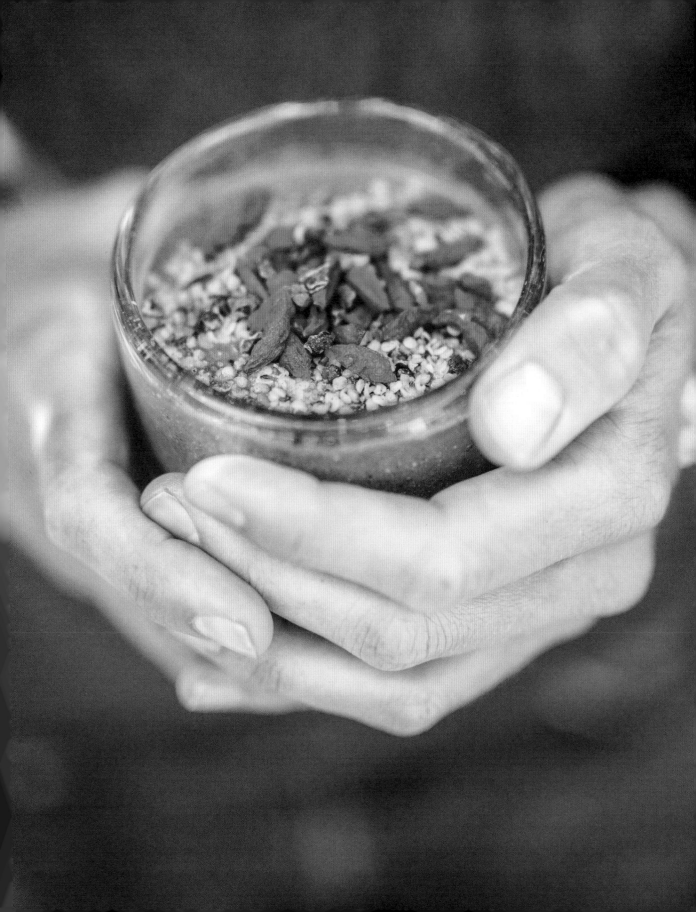

Mango is magic. It's a great low-calorie food that makes you feel full, while the fibre helps your digestive system, which in turn helps you burn more calories. It is also rich in vitamin A, with one serving giving you 25 per cent of your required daily intake.

MANGO MAGIC

250ml coconut milk

1 tbsp raw honey

1 tbsp coconut oil

1 tbsp chia seeds

1 tsp sunflower seeds

1 tsp flaxseeds

2 tbsp almond butter

2.5cm piece of fresh root ginger, peeled and chopped

1 mango, peeled and destoned

a handful of chopped frozen pineapple

Wash, peel and chop the ingredients where necessary. Put all the ingredients into a blender in the order they're listed. Blitz until smooth.

JUICEMAN FACT
Raw honey has not been heated, pasteurized or processed in any way. It's an alkaline food and is a powerhouse of vitamins, enzymes and antioxidants.

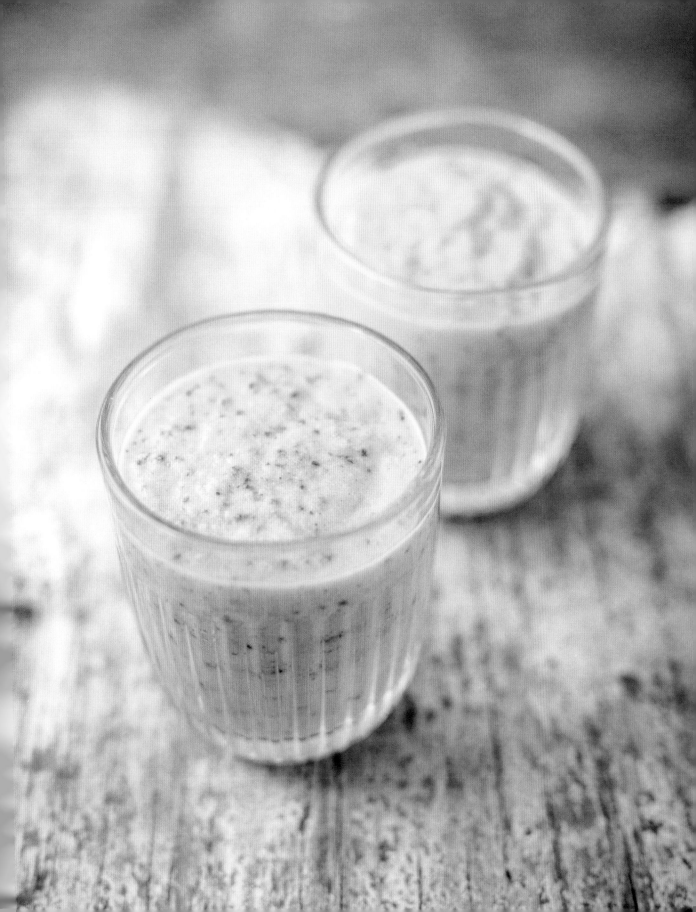

THE GREEN GOD

An amazing smoothie for the morning or to help you get through the day. I have given the option to use kefir in this recipe, as I am a big fan of it. Kefir is a cultured milk drink that is enzyme-rich and filled with friendly microorganisms to help balance your 'inner ecosystem'. It is more nutritious than yogurt and provides complete protein, essential minerals and valuable B vitamins. You can either buy it or make it yourself.

200ml almond or coconut milk

100g coconut yogurt or kefir

1 tsp raw honey or maple syrup

1 tbsp natural protein powder

1 tsp shelled hemp seeds

1 tsp ground flaxseeds

1 tsp pumpkin seeds

a handful of spinach leaves

1 frozen banana

a handful of ice cubes

Wash, peel and chop the ingredients where necessary. Put all the ingredients into a blender in the order they're listed. Blitz until smooth.

JUICEMAN TIP
Add a handful of kale to get your phyto goodness.

GREEN WARRIOR

This one is a fantastic post-workout smoothie, or at any time of the day when you need a power boost. I love to make a double portion of this in the morning to get me through the day.

375ml coconut water

1 tbsp natural protein powder

a pinch of cayenne pepper

a pinch of ground cinnamon

1 tsp flaxseeds

a few sprigs of coriander

1 Medjool date, pitted, or a handful of raisins

½ a lime, peeled

½ a cucumber, chopped

a handful of baby spinach leaves

1 apple, cored and chopped

1 frozen banana

Wash, peel and chop the ingredients where necessary. Put all the ingredients into a blender in the order they're listed. Blitz until smooth.

JUICEMAN TIP
Swap the coconut water for green tea or yerba maté for an extra energy boost after a workout.

HURRICANE

So this is the mother of all smoothies. It will give you a huge power punch, so it's perfect for pre- and post-training, or just when you are in need of a boost. Please don't be put off by the powders – they can all be easily bought and will give your body lots of nutrition. Activated barley is used to boost performance, enhance the immune system and maintain endurance. It is a slow-burning carbohydrate that provides a steady source of energy for long workouts or periods of intense concentration.

325ml coconut water

1 tsp activated barley powder

1 tbsp maca powder

1 tsp chlorella powder

½ a lemon, peeled

1 lime, peeled

a small sprig of parsley

a handful of kale leaves

2 oranges, peeled

¼ of a chopped frozen pineapple

Wash, peel and chop the ingredients where necessary. Put all the ingredients into a blender in the order they're listed. Blitz until smooth.

JUICEMAN FACT
The Roman army marched on a diet of barley!

CHOCOLATE POWER SHAKE

This is my go-to-after-the-gym shake. It's a real treat to look forward to after a tough workout. My wife always steals it from me, gym or not, so it must taste good.

350ml almond milk or coconut water

2 tbsp natural protein powder

a pinch of vanilla powder

a pinch of ground cinnamon

1 tbsp raw cacao powder or nibs

1 tbsp chia seeds

1 tsp flaxseeds

1 Medjool date, pitted

1 frozen banana

Wash, peel and chop the ingredients where necessary. Put all the ingredients into a blender in the order they're listed. Blitz until smooth.

JUICEMAN TIPS
If you are feeling adventurous, add some deer antler velvet for muscle-tissue repair. It is known to increase growth hormones and keep you looking young for longer. Chocolate-flavoured protein powder works really well here.

Protein is an important part of everyone's diet. I love to use vanilla-flavoured protein powder in this one but feel free to use your favourite. For anyone who isn't a fan of cacao, this is a pink version of my Chocolate Power Shake (see p.91). It's definitely just as delicious!

PINK POWER SHAKE

250ml coconut water

150ml nut milk of your choice

1 tbsp natural protein powder

a pinch of vanilla powder

1 tsp goji berries

2 tsp chia seeds

1 tbsp almond butter

1 Medjool date, pitted

2 handfuls of frozen strawberries

Wash, peel and chop the ingredients where necessary. Put all the ingredients into a blender in the order they're listed. Blitz until smooth.

JUICEMAN TIP
Top with bee pollen and hemp seeds for the beauty factor.

JUICEMAN FACT
Goji berries are known to improve fertility and protect eyesight.

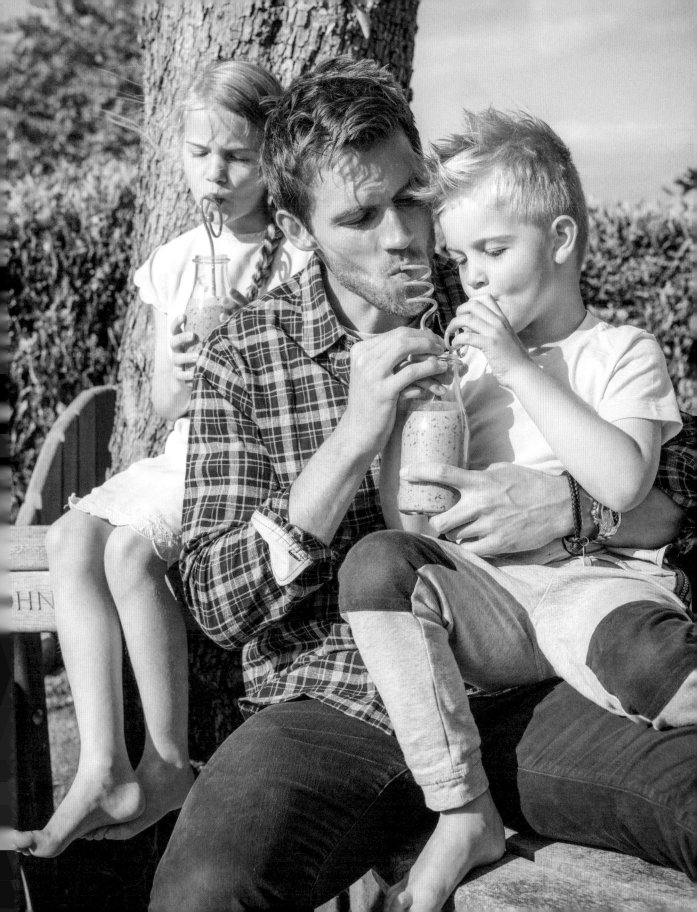

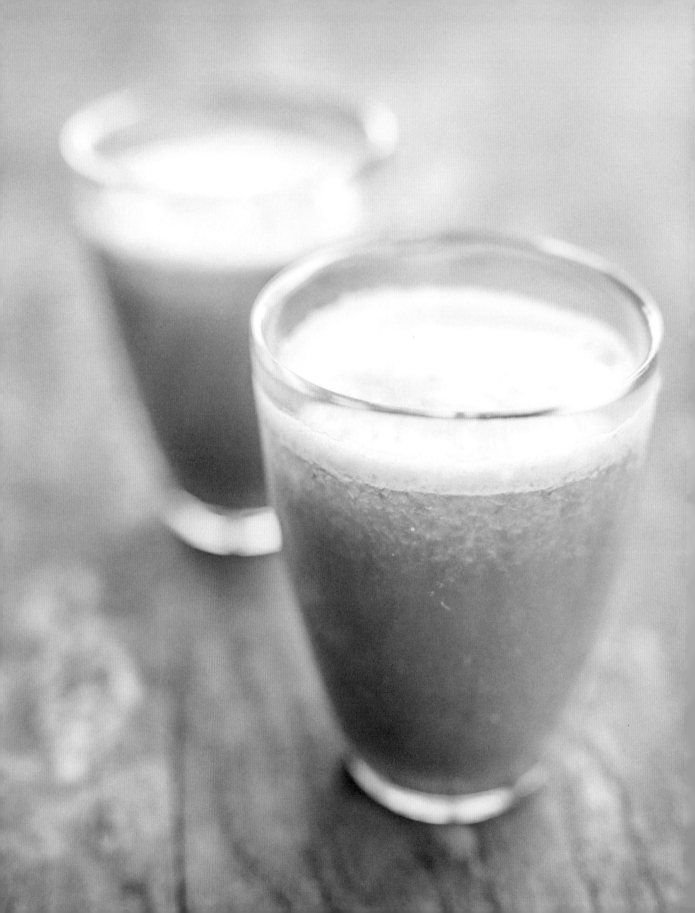

This smoothie will make you feel that you have been very good to your body. Full of nutrient-packed fruit and veg, it will give your system a real boost. I do not peel kiwis, as the skin is full of vitamin C and fibre – perfect for smoothies. As this is a meal in a glass, it is a great way to finish your day.

GREEN GIANT

325ml mineral water or coconut water

1 tsp spirulina

1 tsp maca powder

1 tsp flaxseeds

1 tsp coconut or hemp oil

a sprig of parsley

a handful of kale leaves

2.5cm piece of fresh root ginger, peeled

2 kiwi fruits, chopped

a handful of baby spinach leaves

½ a lemon, peeled

½ a cucumber, chopped

Wash, peel and chop the ingredients where necessary. Put all the ingredients into a blender in the order they're listed. Blitz until smooth.

JUICEMAN TIP
Top with coconut flakes and goji berries for an extra immunity boost.

JUICEMAN FACT
Maca boosts sex drive.

TROPICAL THUNDER

My kids love this recipe because it is really creamy and sweet. There are tons of superfoods that are great for putting in smoothies. Goji berries are one of my favourites, as they are the most nutrient-rich fruit on the planet. They also taste delicious, so throw them into everything if you can.

350ml coconut milk

a pinch of vanilla powder

a small handful of goji berries

1 Medjool date, pitted, or 1 tsp raw honey

1 chopped frozen mango

a handful of frozen strawberries

1 frozen banana

Wash, peel and chop the ingredients where necessary. Put all the ingredients into a blender in the order they're listed. Blitz until smooth.

JUICEMAN TIP
Throw in some spinach or kale for extra chlorophyll goodness.

JUICEMAN FACT
Vanilla contains high levels of antioxidants so it can help you to stay looking young.

PICK-ME-UP

Had a late night? If you're feeling sluggish and are in need of a pick-me-up, this is the smoothie for you. The benefit of using yerba mate tea in this one is that it is a natural stimulant with the strength of coffee and the health benefits of tea, delivering both energy and nutrition.

350ml coconut water or yerba maté tea

1 tsp chia seeds

2 slices of fresh root turmeric, peeled or 1 tsp ground turmeric powder

1 lemon, peeled

1 orange, peeled

2 carrots, chopped

Wash, peel and chop the ingredients where necessary. Put all the ingredients into a blender in the order they're listed. Blitz until smooth.

JUICEMAN FACT
Yerba maté is traditionally used as an appetite suppressant and to help with weight loss.

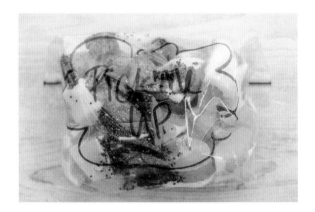

GREEN BANGKOK

A flavourful, exotic smoothie for any occasion. I love all these beautiful ingredients mixed together. It is wonderful to drink at any time of day, especially when the sun is shining.

250ml coconut water

1 tsp coconut oil or butter

½ a red or green chilli

2.5cm piece of fresh root ginger, peeled and chopped

1 Medjool date, pitted

½ a lime, peeled

a small bunch of coriander

½ a celery stick

¼ of a cucumber, chopped

a handful of baby spinach leaves

½ a chopped frozen pineapple

a handful of ice cubes

Wash, peel and chop the ingredients where necessary. Put all the ingredients into a blender in the order they're listed. Blitz until smooth.

JUICEMAN FACT
Pineapple contains bromelain, which is an anti-inflammatory and helps digestion.

DIET SMOOTHIE

Not only is this a really tasty smoothie, it's also great for anyone on a weight-loss programme. Foods that are high in fibre or water content, or both, help to create a lasting feeling of fullness, while being very low in calories. This smoothie is also perfect for satisfying a sweet tooth.

½ a watermelon, peeled and chopped

1 lemon, peeled

1 tsp raw honey

Wash, peel and chop the ingredients where necessary. Put all the ingredients into a blender in the order they're listed. Blitz until smooth.

JUICEMAN FACT
Watermelon is a great source of lycopene, which is known to help prevent cancer.

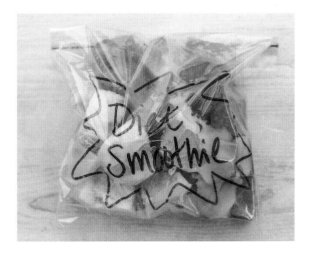

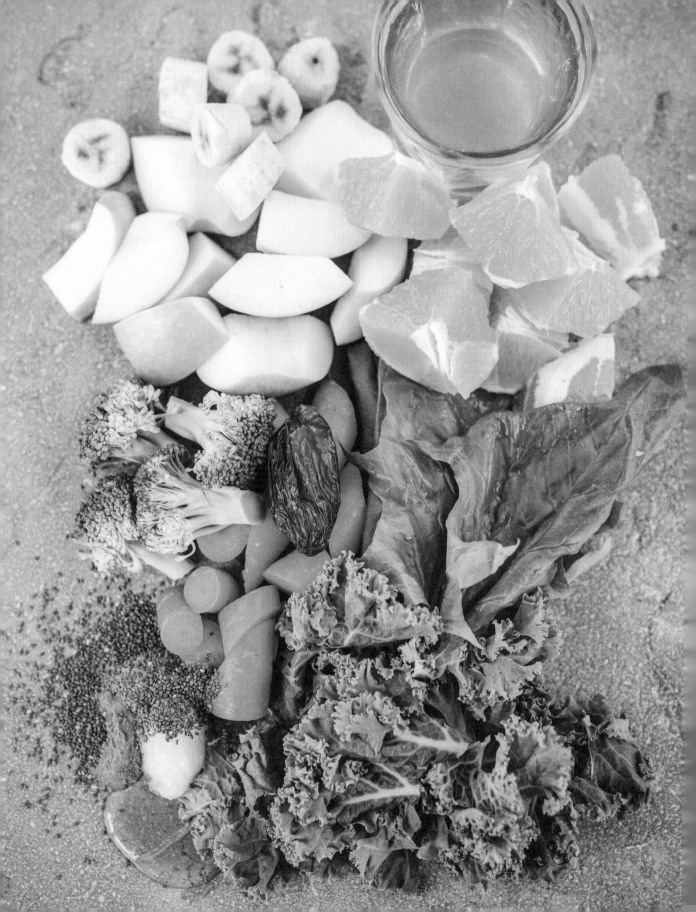

I love all the colours when I'm prepping this smoothie. There are so many amazing ingredients to help give your immune system a boost. Make this one for a friend and then ask them to guess what's in it. They'll never get it right, but I guarantee that they will like it.

THE SECRET SMOOTHIE

500ml mineral water or coconut water

a pinch of ground cinnamon

1 tsp chia seeds

1 tsp coconut oil

1 tsp raw honey

1 Medjool date, pitted

1 apple, cored and chopped

4 small broccoli florets

1 carrot, chopped

1 orange, peeled

a handful of spinach leaves

a handful of roughly chopped kale or chard leaves

1 frozen banana

Wash, peel and chop the ingredients where necessary. Put all the ingredients into a blender in the order they're listed. Blitz until smooth.

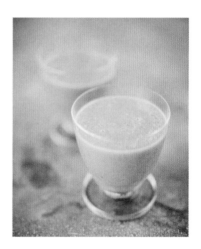

While I was filming *The Royals*, I would make this with my co-star Alexandra Park as she is a Type 1 diabetic. This is the ultimate in supercharged smoothies without the sugar. Warning: this one is not for the faint-hearted. You will either love it or hate it. It's the ultimate all-veg green smoothie.

THE ROYAL GREEN

500ml coconut water

1 tsp spirulina

1 tsp chlorella powder

a pinch of ground cinnamon

a pinch of cayenne pepper

1 tsp chaga mushroom

2.5cm piece of fresh root turmeric, peeled

2.5cm piece of fresh root ginger, peeled and chopped

1 lemon, peeled

1 cucumber, chopped

2 celery sticks, chopped

a bunch of coriander

a handful of kale leaves

Wash, peel and chop the ingredients where necessary. Put all the ingredients into a blender in the order they're listed. Blitz until smooth.

After a hard workout your muscles need to recover, and a smoothie with ingredients that are known to have anti-inflammatory benefits is just what your body needs. If you train hard to look good on the outside, this drink will help look after everything you need inside. I like using hemp protein powder for this one.

REPAIR AND REBOOT

300ml mineral water or coconut water

1 tbsp natural protein powder

1 tsp flaxseeds

1 tbsp pumpkin seeds

2.5cm piece of fresh root turmeric, peeled, or ½ tsp ground turmeric

2.5cm piece of fresh root ginger, peeled and chopped

¼ of a frozen chopped pineapple

1 frozen banana

a handful of ice cubes

Wash, peel and chop the ingredients where necessary. Put all the ingredients into a blender in the order they're listed. Blitz until smooth.

JUICEMAN FACT
Pumpkin seeds are high in zinc, which is important for strong hair and nails.

This is so easy and quick to make, and it really hits the spot after a workout. It will help to restore your energy and strength, which leads to a fast recovery. You can use any protein powder, but a vanilla one works well with the bananas to give a great-tasting smoothie.

MATCHA RECOVERY SHAKE

350ml almond or cashew milk

1 tbsp natural protein powder

1 tsp matcha green tea powder

2 frozen bananas

Sieve the matcha powder into the milk and mix until no clumps remain. Then combine all the ingredients in a blender and blitz until smooth.

JUICEMAN TIP
Try adding some cacao nibs for extra energy, extra antioxidants and extra crunch. Cacao is also known to elevate your mood.

JUICEMAN FACT
During exercise your body loses potassium through sweat. Eating a banana boosts your potassium levels and gives you 10 per cent of the recommended daily intake.

This smoothie is delicious, and just what you need after a workout. Cherries are known as one of nature's true healing foods. They're packed with antioxidants and offer many health benefits, including help with insomnia, joint pain and belly fat.

CHERRY ON THE TOP

400ml coconut water or the water and meat from a fresh coconut

1 tsp lucuma powder

150g frozen pitted cherries

a handful of spinach leaves

1 frozen banana

Wash, peel and chop the ingredients where necessary. Put all the ingredients into a blender in the order they're listed. Blitz until smooth.

JUICEMAN TIP
Remember to take the stones out of the cherries before freezing.

JUICEMAN FACT
Cherries contain melatonin, which can aid sleep, so have a handful before bed for a good night's zzzzzz.

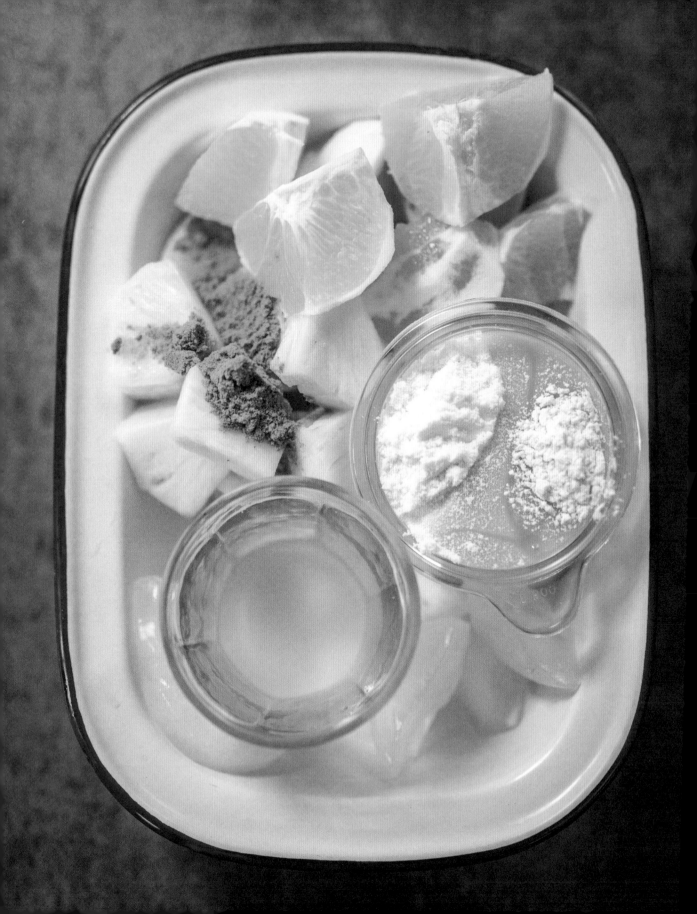

To have good overall health, you need a healthy gut and digestion. Perm A vite Powder is a product I use a lot. It provides large amounts of cellulose fibre and L-glutamine, with additional nutrients including N-acetyl-D-glucosamine, slippery elm bark and MSM. Don't be put off by the long words; it basically helps look after your gut, which is like your body's second brain, so it's really important. It has helped me in so many ways!

BE GOOD TO YOURSELF

250ml coconut water

2 tbsp natural protein powder

1 tsp Perm A vite Powder or L-glutamine powder

1 tsp ground turmeric

1 tsp manuka honey

2 oranges, peeled

¼ of a chopped frozen pineapple

a handful of ice cubes

Wash, peel and chop the ingredients where necessary. Put all the ingredients into a blender in the order they're listed. Blitz until smooth.

JUICEMAN FACT
L-glutamine is key for post-workout recovery and hugely beneficial for your digestive system.

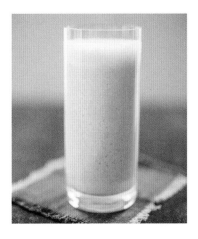

This is great for people needing to reboot after a gym session – a tasty, refreshing drink that gives you a super-kick of energy. It also works well as a meal replacement. I love hemp, and this one contains hemp oil and I suggest you use hemp protein for your protein powder here too. The hemp seed is bursting with omega-6 and omega-3, essential fatty acids that are known to have heart-health and anti-inflammatory benefits.

RAGING BULL

300ml coconut water

1 tbsp natural
protein powder

1 tsp maca powder

1 tsp chia seeds

1 tsp pumpkin seeds

1 tsp coconut oil or
coconut butter

1 tsp hemp oil

1 tbsp raw honey

4 Medjool dates, pitted

1 lime, peeled

1 lemon, peeled

1 orange, peeled

Wash, peel and chop the ingredients where necessary. Put all the ingredients into a blender in the order they're listed. Blitz until smooth.

JUICEMAN FACT
The vitamin C in the citrus fruits will help your body absorb the iron from the pumpkin seeds, which have one of the highest iron contents of any seed.

Close your eyes when you drink this one and you could be sunning yourself in a beautiful tropical paradise. These ingredients do make me think of holidaying in the Caribbean, but why not drink it all year round? If you keep all the ingredients frozen, you can have it any time!

MANGO PUNCH

250ml almond milk

1 tbsp flaxseeds

2 tbsp hemp seeds

¼ of a jalapeño chilli, chopped

1 lime, peeled

a large handful of chopped frozen mango

¼ of a chopped frozen pineapple

½ a frozen banana

Wash, peel and chop the ingredients where necessary. Put all the ingredients into a blender in the order they're listed. Blitz until smooth.

JUICEMAN TIPS
Top with flaked coconut for a truly tropical experience. Add a shot of rum for a delicious cocktail.

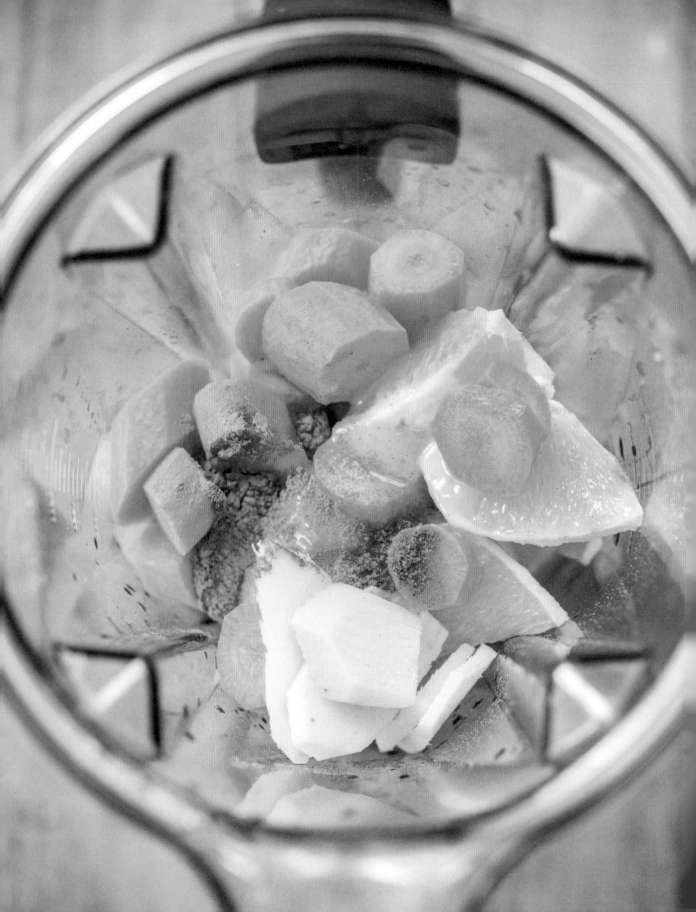

This is a good example of how you can make your favourite juice ingredients into a smoothie. Feeling a bit run-down, or getting ready for the onset of winter? This has the ingredients to give you a big immune boost, which will help you fight off colds and illness.

FLU JAB

250ml mineral water

a pinch of ground cinnamon

a pinch of cayenne pepper

1 tbsp manuka honey

2.5cm piece of fresh root ginger, peeled and chopped

½ a lemon, peeled

1 apple, cored and chopped

1 orange, peeled

2 carrots, chopped

Wash, peel and chop the ingredients where necessary. Put all the ingredients into a blender in the order they're listed. Blitz until smooth.

JUICEMAN TIP
For extra health benefits add 10 drops of echinacea.

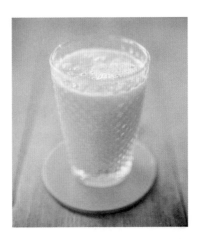

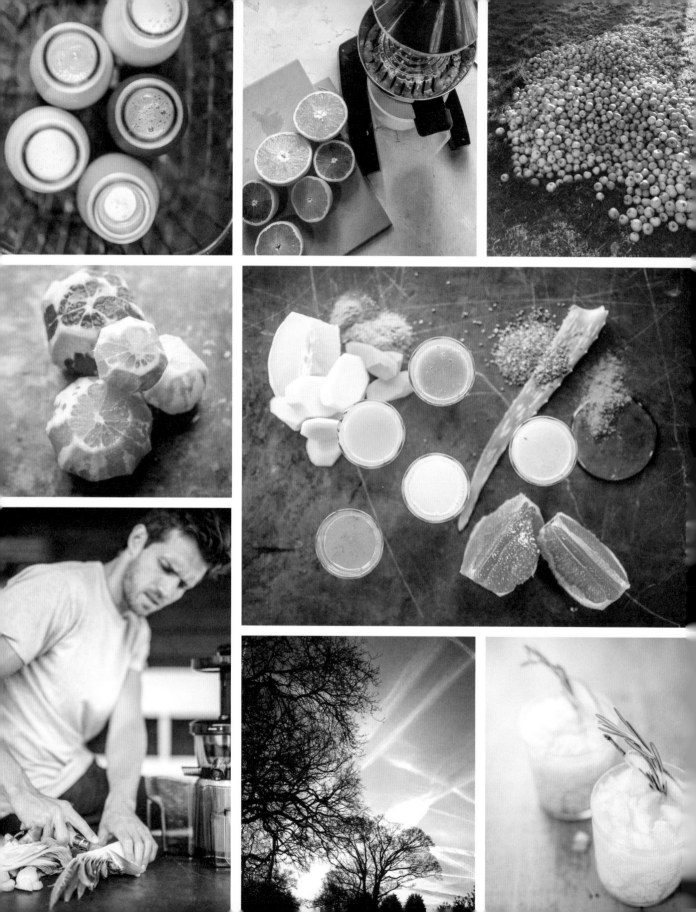

SHOTS AND TONICS

Shots are addictive. They are now something I do every time I use my juicer. They are quick and easy and you can create the most awesome nutrient-rich, medicinal fireballs, not to mention you can use them in loads of different ways.

At the Juiceman factory, shots are my favourite thing to play with and there is nothing better than the smell of fresh-pressed ginger and lemon. A word of warning though . . . pure ginger is not for the faint-hearted, so go easy and start by pairing it with celery or apple.

When I have a cold coming on, I am straight in with the fresh ginger, lemon and honey with warm water (see p.116). You can also freeze a bulk load of shots in ice cube trays. These can then be defrosted and drunk neat or simply added to water.

I like to use shots with water to make tonics. Why not try adding your ginger, turmeric and lemon shot to some cold water for a health tonic on a hot day or after a gym session. Have fun and play around with the flavour and heat . . .

All recipes serve 1.

The name says it all. Make it when you need it!
This is great as a shot or tonic, and brilliant for
when you're feeling run-down.

GET WELL

½ an orange, peeled

5cm piece of fresh
root ginger

1 slice of chilli

1 tsp colloidal silver

1 tsp echinacea powder

Juice the orange, ginger and chilli, then mix
with the other ingredients. Serve straight up,
or in 300–500ml of warm water or cold water
with ice.

JUICEMAN TIP
A friend of mine recommended the brand
MesoSilver, which claims to be a true colloidal
silver. We use it whenever anyone in the family
is coming down with a cold.

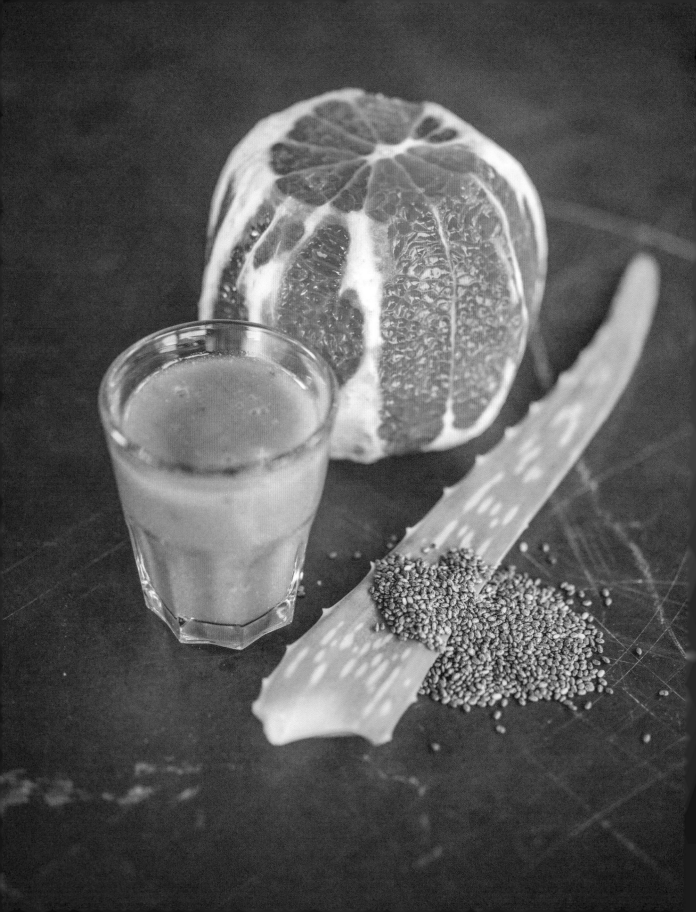

My sister loves this shot. It takes a little time to prepare, but using a fresh aloe leaf is definitely the way forward. Aloe vera is the bomb. It's really easy to grow and easy to drink when mixed with grapefruit juice.

SKIN SHOT

1 grapefruit, peeled

1 aloe vera leaf, peeled

½ a cucumber

1 tsp chia seeds

Blitz the grapefruit, inner aloe vera gel and cucumber in a blender until smooth, then add the chia seeds, stir and leave in the fridge for 10 minutes before enjoying.

JUICEMAN TIP
To peel the aloe vera leaf, lie it flat and remove the sides. Then run a knife under the top and bottom outer layers, as if you're filleting a fish.

MORNING SHOT

This is my daily ritual. The lemon and ginger helps waken your body and digestive system, while also alkalising your body and invigorating your metabolism. I enjoy mine with warm water.

1 lemon peeled	5cm piece of fresh root ginger, peeled

Juice the ingredients and serve straight up, or in 300–500ml of warm water or cold water with ice.

JUICEMAN TIP
I like to add 1 teaspoon of manuka honey if I feel like something a bit sweeter.

SOS

I love turmeric for its incredible healing properites. This is a great shot – and it's even better as a tonic. Mix with water at 10 parts water to 1 part shot, and enjoy after a run or yoga session.

5cm piece of fresh root ginger, peeled	1 tsp coconut sugar
2.5cm piece of fresh root turmeric, peeled	a pinch of ground cinnamon
½ a lemon, peeled	

Juice the ingredients and serve straight up, or in 300–500ml of warm water or cold water with ice.

JUICEMAN TIP
Make sure you drink a glass of water after consuming turmeric to avoid any teeth staining.

TUMMY TUCK

If you don't know about apple cider vinegar then let's just start by saying it's amazing and has unbelievable healing qualities. Make sure you buy one that contains the 'mother' – strands of proteins, enzymes and friendly bacteria that give the product a murky, cobweb-like appearance. I love this shot as it helps to settle my stomach, and it's also great to help boost your immune system.

1 tsp apple cider vinegar	a pinch of ground cayenne pepper
1 tsp raw honey	a pinch of ground cinnamon

Juice the ingredients and serve straight up, or in 300–500ml warm water or cold water with ice.

RAW HEAT

This shot can be as big as needed and is my go-to when I'm starting to feel a bit run-down or like I'm getting a cold. It's great for clearing your sinuses, and celery is also super-alkaline and detoxifying.

2 celery sticks	5cm piece of fresh root ginger
½ a lemon, peeled	

Juice the ingredients and serve straight up, or in 300–500ml of warm water or cold water with ice.

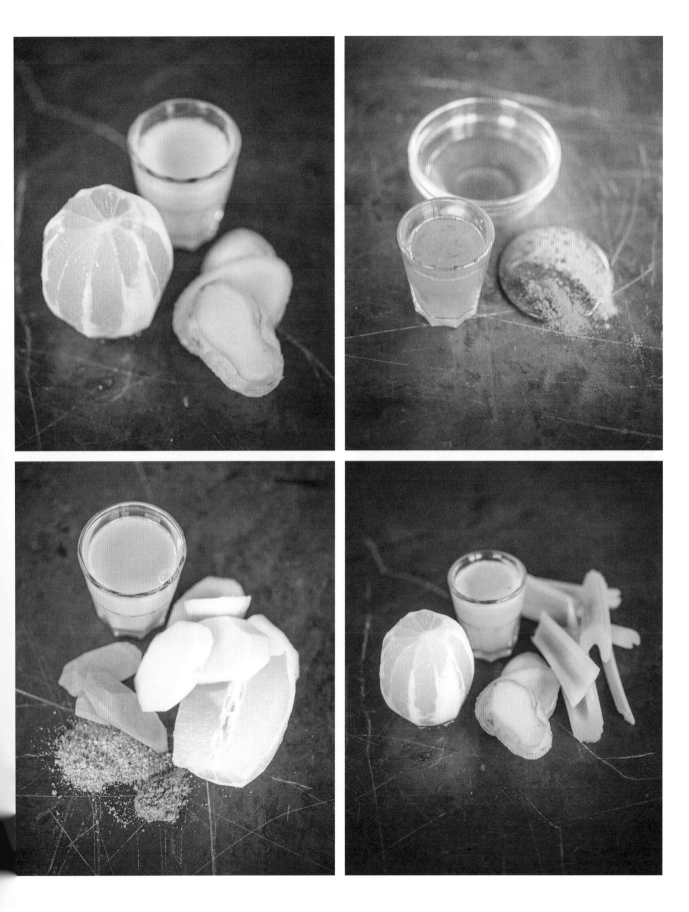

This makes a great shot, but I prefer it with the added water (see photo) to make a rehydrating drink that's perfect for yoga or post-workout. It contains some Indian flavours and is a great shade of orange. Remember to peel the turmeric with care . . .

YOGA SHOT

5cm piece of fresh root ginger, peeled

2.5cm piece of fresh root turmeric, peeled

½ a lemon, peeled

1 tsp coconut sugar

a pinch of Himalayan salt

a pinch of ground cinnamon

a pinch of ground cardamom

a pinch of black pepper

Juice the ginger, turmeric and lemon, then mix with the other ingredients and serve straight up or in 300–500ml of warm water or cold water with ice.

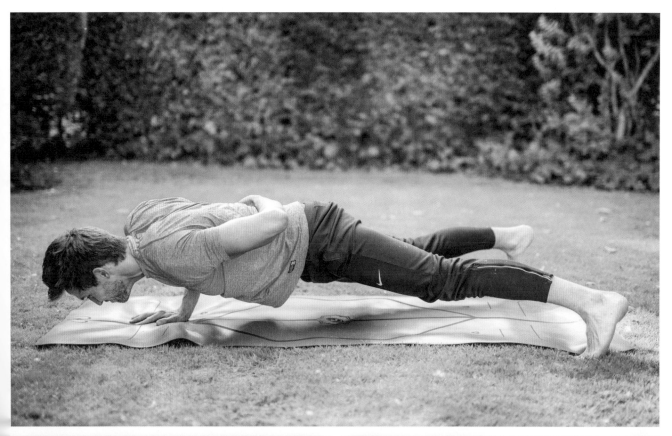

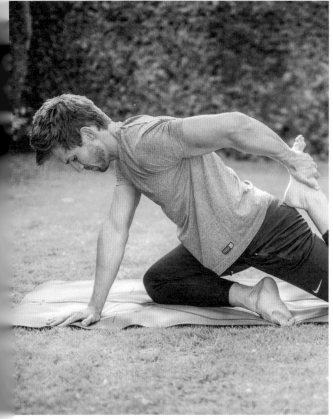

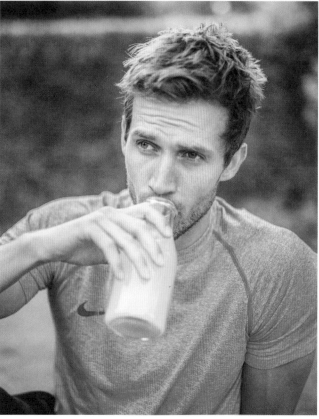

Whenever I'm looking to detox, I add one of these shots to my daily routine. Activated charcoal is a must for those looking to cleanse. This amazing black powder helps to draw out toxins and impurities from your system. Don't be put off by how it looks! It's easy to drink and doesn't taste of much at all.

ACTIVATED CHARCOAL TONIC

1 tsp activated charcoal

1 tsp coconut sugar or maple syrup

juice of ½ a lemon

500ml mineral water

Simply mix the ingredients together and enjoy.

JUICEMAN TIP
Drink this between meals on an empty stomach for maximum benefit. It's also an old-school cure for food poisoning and toxicity.

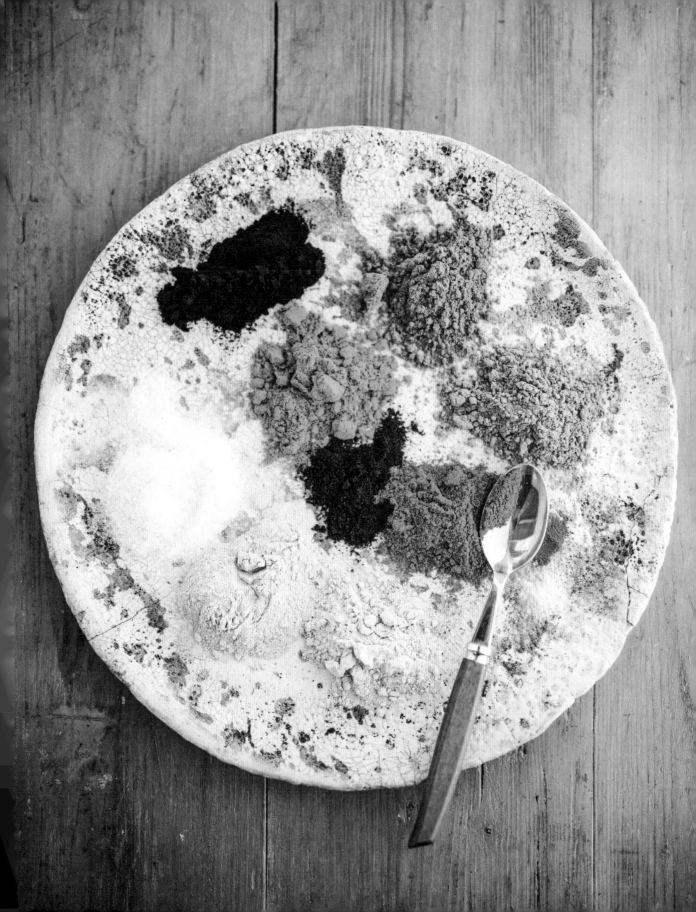

FIREBALL)))

I highly recommend adding oregano oil to your arsenal of natural healing tools, as it has a wide range of uses. This herbal oil is a powerful antimicrobial that can help fight off infections. Oregano oil also has antibacterial, antiviral and antifungal properties. This recipe is a great hangover cure. It will clear your head, but beware: it will be hot!

1 orange, peeled

5cm piece of fresh root ginger

a pinch of cayenne pepper or 1 slice of hot red chilli

2 drops of oregano oil

Juice the orange and ginger, then mix in the cayenne pepper (or chilli, if using) and oregano oil. Serve straight up or in 300–500ml of warm water or cold water with ice.

THE HEALER

MSM is a key source of sulphur and is a staple in my diet. It has a series of healing and preventative properties for the human body and is important for bone and joint care, as well as skin and hair care.

¼ of a cucumber

½ a lemon, peeled

1 tsp MSM powder

1 tsp aloe vera juice

Juice the cucumber and lemon, then mix with the remaining ingredients and serve straight up.

JUICEMAN FACT
MSM is often referred to as the 'beauty supplement' because of its ability to enhance the thickness of hair and strength of nails in a very short time frame.

BRAIN BOOSTER

Coriander is one of the very few herbs that is used as a heavy-metal detox agent to detoxify mercury, aluminium and lead, among others. I often make a small bottle of neat, concentrated coriander juice and mix it with chlorella powder. Drink a shot of this booster every day and feel the improvement to your brain power.

a small bunch of coriander

½ an apple

½ a lemon, peeled

1 tsp chlorella powder

Juice the coriander, apple and lemon, then add the chlorella powder and serve straight up.

LAST RESORT

All my favourite powerful ingredients in one very small package. It may not be a pleasure to drink, but it will do the job and give you a huge boost. Good luck!

1 garlic clove

2.5cm piece of fresh root ginger, peeled

1 tbsp aloe vera juice

1 drop of oregano oil

a pinch of cayenne pepper

2 drops of echinacea

Juice the garlic and ginger, then add the remaining ingredients and serve straight up.

JUICEMAN FACT
Cayenne pepper boosts the metabolism.

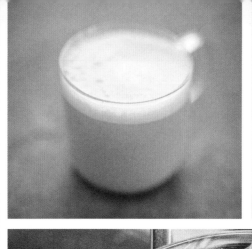

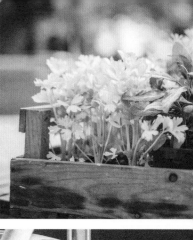

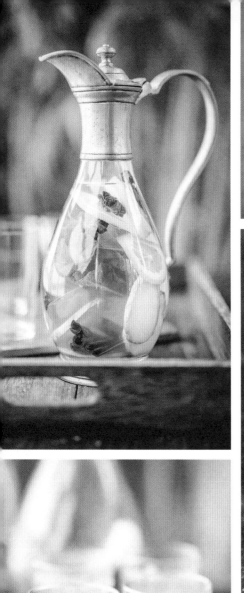

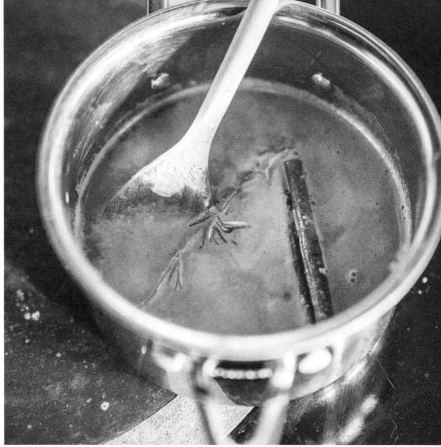

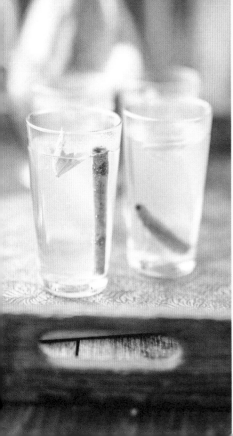

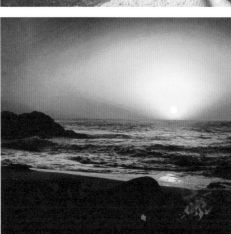

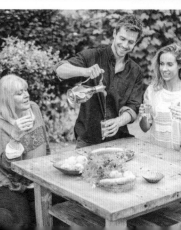

TEAS AND
WARM DRINKS

Natural teas are another great way to incorporate fresh fruit or many of your store cupboard ingredients into your daily routine. It amazes me how many people now drink warm water every morning to rebalance and alkalize their system. Don't stop there! Try adding herbs, spices, citrus fruits, or even some of the shots from pages 112–23.

One of my favourite ingredients is apple cider vinegar. It's unbelievably good for you and is one of the oldest natural cures for a whole range of ailments. I particularly enjoy it in warm water with some cinnamon and raw honey.

My tip would be to invest in a good-quality loose-leaf teapot so you can play with your infusions.

Apple cider vinegar is an important part of my daily routine – whether it's in salad dressings, teas or a morning shot. This is my winter flu-fighting drink when I'm feeling fatigued or under the weather. It is also great to have before a big meal as it aids digestion.

HOT CIDER HEALER

500ml warm water

1 tbsp apple cider vinegar

1 tsp ground cinnamon

2 slices of fresh root ginger, peeled

1 tsp raw or manuka honey

a pinch of cayenne pepper, optional

Combine all the ingredients together and stir well.

JUICEMAN TIP
If you get a breakout of spots, try dabbing on neat apple cider vinegar . . . It works for me!

JUICEMAN FACT
Apple cider vinegar helps to speed up the metabolism. It also supports fat burning and can control appetite.

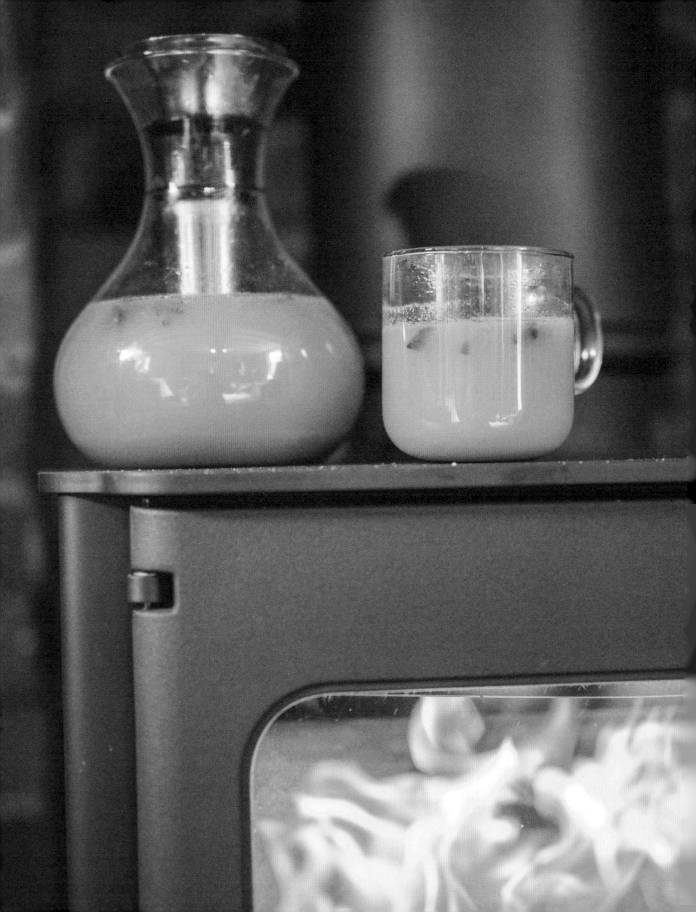

This drink sits between a juice and a soup. I love how the apples/pineapple blend with the carrot and spices.

WARM WINTER SPICE

5 apples or ¼ of a pineapple, peeled and cored

1 orange, peeled

1 cinnamon stick

2 star anise

a sprig of rosemary

4 carrots

2.5cm piece of fresh root ginger, peeled and grated

a pinch of ground cinnamon

a pinch of ground nutmeg

Juice the apples (or the pineapple, if using) and the orange and pour the juice into a saucepan. Add the cinnamon stick, star anise and rosemary, then cover with a lid. Bring to the boil and allow to simmer for 1–2 minutes. Turn off the heat and set aside, covered, for 5 minutes, then strain through a fine sieve.

Juice the carrots and ginger and mix with the warm spiced apple juice. Pour into glasses and sprinkle with the cinnamon and nutmeg before serving.

JUICEMAN TIP
Add some rum to turn it into a winter punch.

Matcha is the ultimate green tea as it consists of the whole leaf in powdered form. It can be used like coffee, to make anything from a matcha shot to a matcha cappuccino. This is a delicious, warming tea. With all the goodness from the matcha and almonds, your body will feel comforted, too.

MATCHA LATTE

250ml almond milk

1 tsp matcha green tea powder

a pinch of vanilla powder

To serve hot, place the milk in a pan with the other ingredients and warm over a low heat. Use a whisk to make sure there are no lumps.

JUICEMAN TIP
For extra sweetness, add some manuka honey and then sprinkle some cinnamon on top.

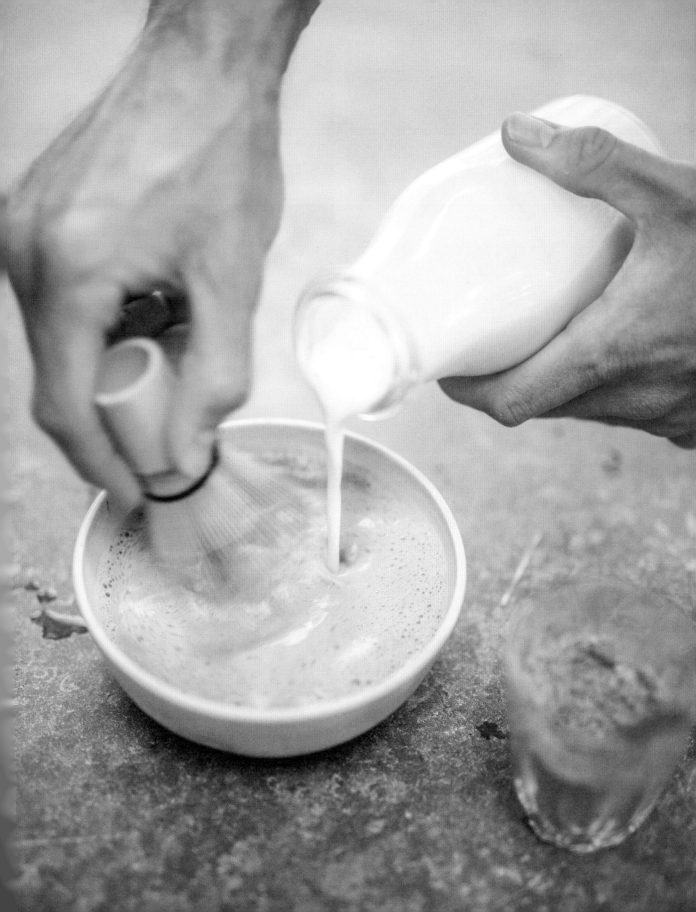

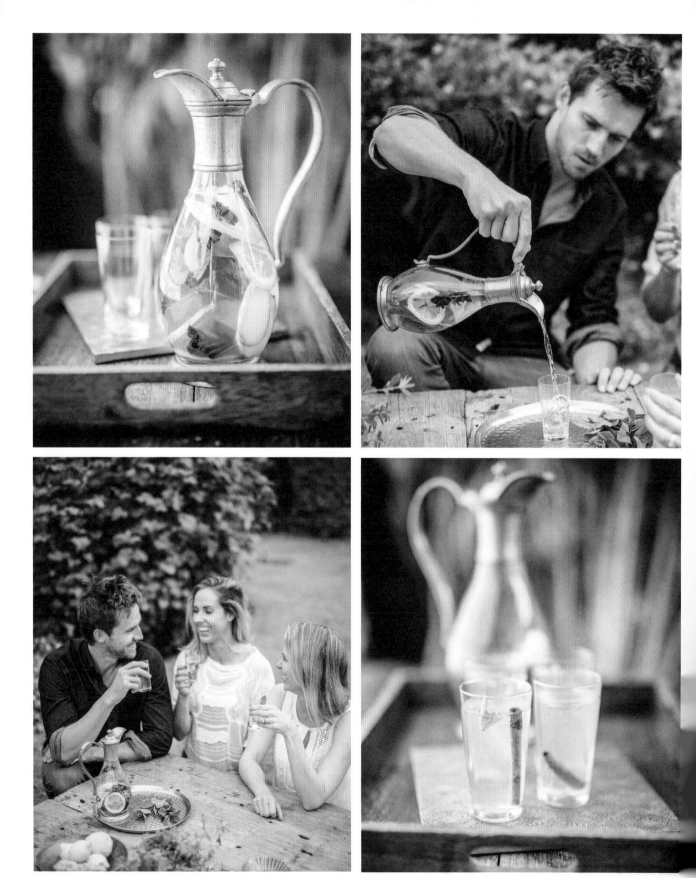

We all know how good mint tea is at the end of a meal to aid digestion, but don't just save it for after you've eaten – this tea will make you feel refreshed at any time of day. If you have any leftovers, strain and store in a glass bottle in the fridge.

MOROCCAN MINT TEA

½ a lemon, peeled

a small handful of mint leaves

1 cinnamon stick

1 star anise

manuka honey, to taste

1 slice of fresh root ginger

Slice the lemon and place in a large cup. Add the mint leaves, then crush them to get the aromas going. Next, add the cinnamon and star anise. Pour over freshly boiled water. Steep the tea for 5 minutes. Enjoy with a little manuka honey and add a slither of ginger.

JUICEMAN TIP
Double the ingredients and place in a pot for more than one serving. You can keep refreshing this with water or use the leftovers in a smoothie – just remember to remove the spices.

This is how I start my day and it feels both refreshing and invigorating. The cayenne pepper is excellent for getting your digestive system fired up, the maple syrup is for energy and the lemon is to cleanse.

TEATOX

½ a lemon, peeled

a mug of warm water
(or you can make it with
cold water in the summer)

2.5cm piece of fresh root
ginger, peeled and grated

a pinch of cayenne pepper

1 tsp maple syrup

Slice the lemon and put it into a teapot of water. Add the rest of the ingredients and stir.

JUICEMAN TIP
You can make a batch and keep it in the fridge for 3–5 days or you can freeze it.

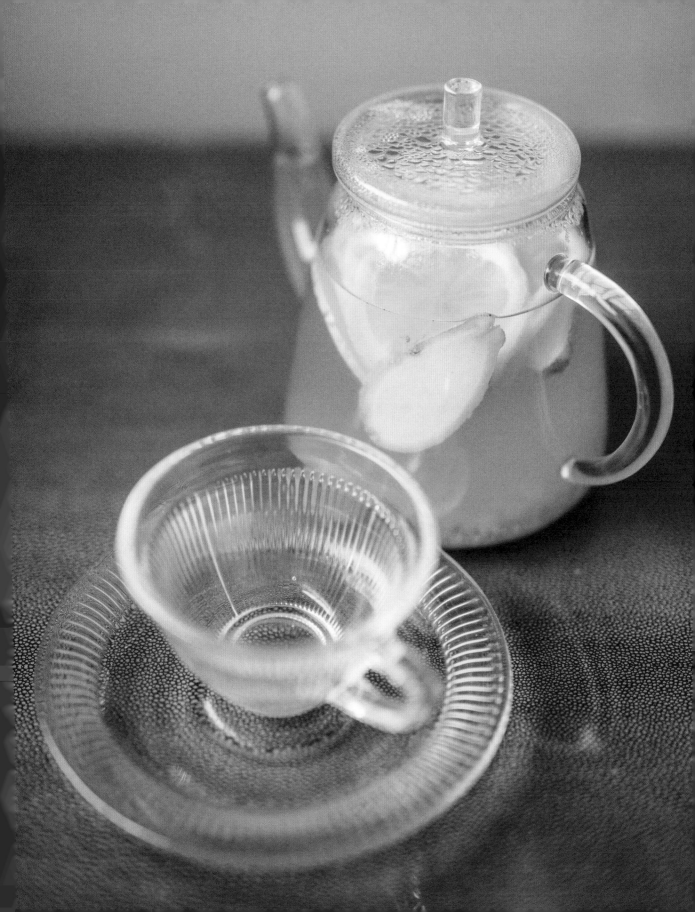

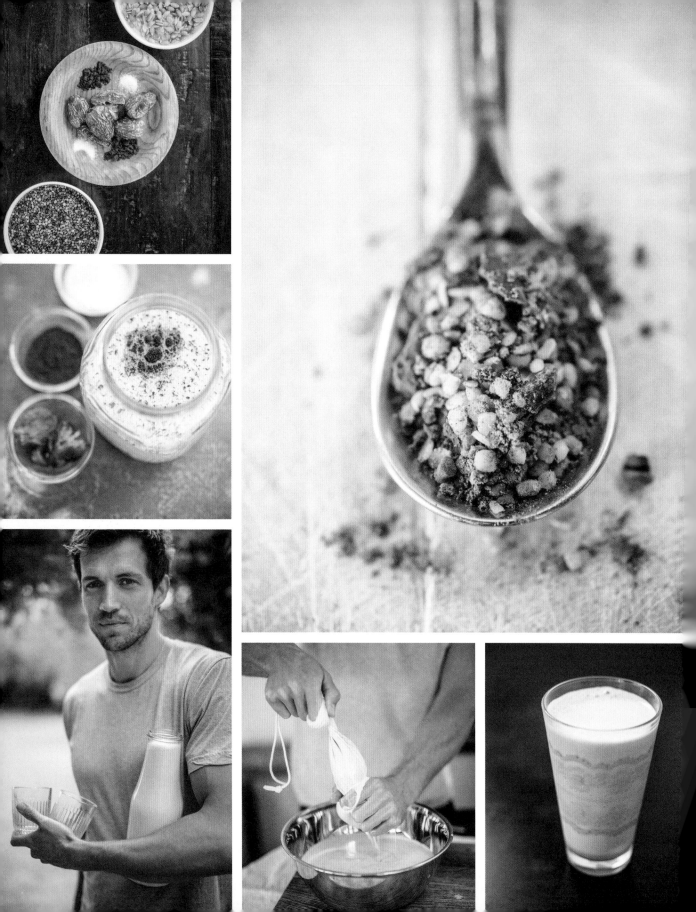

NUT MILKS

There are many views on dairy and milk. I'm gonna give you my two pennies' worth here. Cows' milk is undoubtedly produced to feed calves, which we are not, so it's not a stable nutritional solution for us, even though we are told that a glass a day is good. I do, though, believe that, like butter, it does have beneficial vitamins and has its place in our diet, but that it's not to be consumed in large quantities daily. I also believe in the importance of using organic where possible, to support the humane treatment of cows and the safer production of milk. But enough about that . . . On to the good stuff!

Nut milk is not only delicious and unbelievably nutritious, it's also really easy to make and is a great thing to keep stocked up on for smoothies and breakfasts. It is a staple part of my and my family's daily food and drink – whether it's on porridge, cereal or in a smoothie.

You'll need a nut milk bag for this chapter. A fine sieve will also work well, although you'll end up with a coarser texture.

The recipes in this chapter make 850ml.

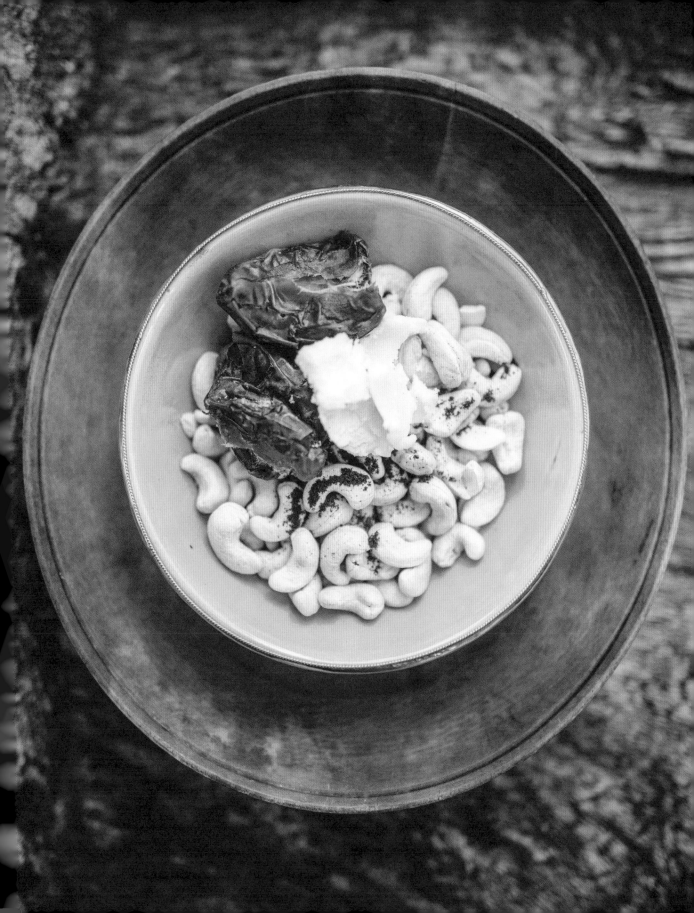

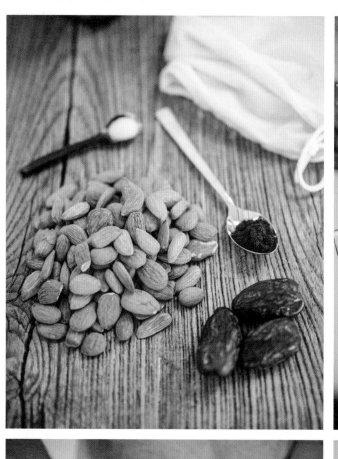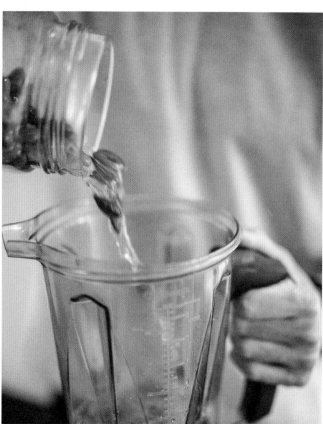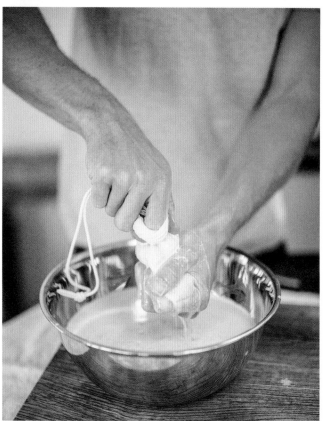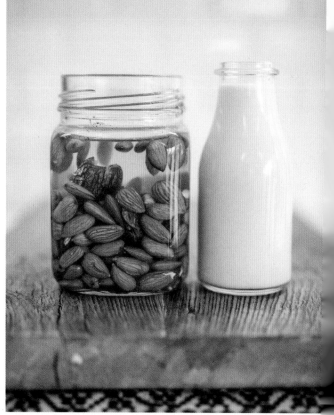

If you were to compare nut milk to dairy milk, almond would be semi-skimmed. Organic almonds have one of the highest nutrient levels of all nuts and, together with the potassium and copper-rich dates, the antioxidant-filled vanilla and alkalizing Himalayan salt, they make a deliciously healthy milk. It can be drunk on its own or used in a whole host of other recipes, including ice cream and smoothies, or on your porridge or granola at breakfast time.

ALMOND MILK

100g almonds

2 Medjool dates, pitted

750ml mineral water

a pinch of vanilla powder

a pinch of Himalayan salt

Equipment: a nut milk bag

Soak the nuts and dates in the water for 6 hours, or overnight, making sure they're well covered.

Place all the ingredients in a blender, including the water the nuts and dates were soaked in. Fill the blender with more water to 850ml. Blend for 1–2 minutes until smooth and creamy, taking care not to let the milk heat up.

Strain through a nut milk bag into a jug or sterilized airtight glass bottles. Refrigerate and use within 3 days.

JUICEMAN TIP
Try adding coconut butter or oil for added energy, or a few pumpkin seeds.

CASHEW MILK

This is the full-cream option of the nut-milk world. It's delicious and creamy, making it a great addition to porridge or smoothies. Cashew nuts are full of vitamin K, copper and magnesium, which are essential for energy, metabolism and nerve function. They are also a great source of good fats, with zero cholesterol, making them the perfect snack.

100g cashew nuts	a pinch of vanilla powder
2 Medjool dates, pitted	a pinch of Himalayan salt
750ml mineral water	Equipment: a nut milk bag

Soak the nuts and dates in the water for 6 hours, or overnight, making sure they're well covered.

Place all the ingredients in a blender, including the water the nuts and dates were soaked in. Fill the blender with more water to 850ml. Blend for 1–2 minutes until smooth and creamy, taking care not to let the milk heat up.

Strain through a fine sieve or nut milk bag into a jug or sterilized airtight glass bottles. Refrigerate and use within 3 days.

JUICEMAN TIP
Try adding turmeric or cinnamon for extra flavour.

Why not try some other variations too? You can simply replace the almonds or cashews in the recipes above with 150g of your favourite nuts or seeds. Here are some suggestions to get you started:

PUMPKIN SEED MILK

Pumpkin seeds are unbelievably good for you on all levels. This milk is rich in zinc, magnesium, iron and omegas, making it great for muscle repair and for general heart and liver health. Play with the sweetness, and possibly add a few nuts to find the right flavour. I love this delicious milk on my porridge.

MACADAMIA NUT MILK

Macadamia nut milk is purely delicious. It has many health and vitality benefits, too, and contains antioxidants such as manganese, vitamin E and zinc. Macadamias also lower your risk of heart disease.

HEMP SEED MILK

Hemp seeds are one of my favourite ingredients, as they are loaded with omega-3 and -6, and are also a great protein source. I like to make this milk and then turn it into a banana and cinnamon shake. Hemp seeds do not need to be soaked.

PISTACHIO NUT MILK

Pistachios are full of B vitamins, copper, manganese, potassium, calcium, iron, magnesium, zinc and selenium. They are also an excellent source of vitamin E. Pistachio milk is a real treat – you have to try it.

BRAZIL NUT MILK

Brazil nuts are a wonderful source of selenium. I like to throw a Brazil nut or two into any shake, just because they are so damn good for you. Brazil nuts do not need to be soaked.

JUICEMAN TIP
Add some raw cacao nibs and carob powder for a Brazil chocolate milkshake.

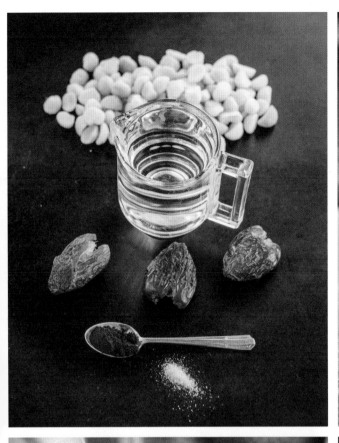

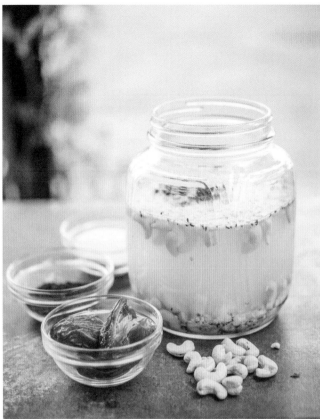

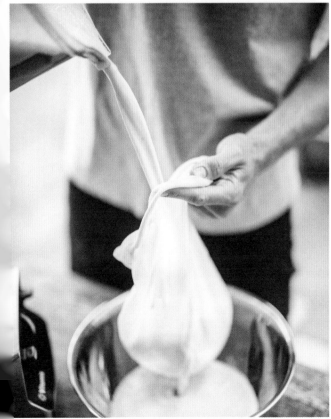

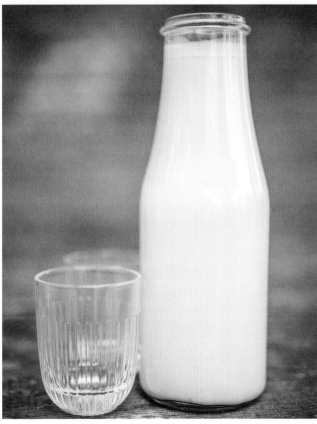

Turmeric is a fantastic natural healer and blends perfectly with cashew milk. I became addicted to turmeric milk in LA at a bar called Moon Juice. I like to drink this milk straight up as a healthy snack. It's a delicious treat that's also great for your body.

TURMERIC MILK

100g cashew nuts

2 Medjool dates, pitted

750ml mineral water

1–2 tsp turmeric powder or 25ml juiced turmeric (peel the turmeric before you juice)

1 tsp raw honey

1 tsp ground cinnamon

a pinch of ground cardamom

a pinch of Himalayan salt

Soak the nuts and dates in the water for 6 hours, or overnight, making sure they're well covered.

Place all the ingredients in a blender, including the water that the nuts and dates were soaked in. Fill the blender with more water to 850ml. Blend for 1–2 minutes until smooth and creamy, taking care not to let the milk heat up.

Strain through a fine sieve or nut milk bag into a jug or sterilized airtight glass bottles. Refrigerate and use within 3 days.

JUICEMAN TIP
Turmeric can stain clothing so be careful when straining the milk.

JUICEMAN FACT
Turmeric is a powerful anti-inflammatory and a strong antioxidant. It's quite hard for us to absorb though, so try swallowing a few whole peppercorns too as this can help.

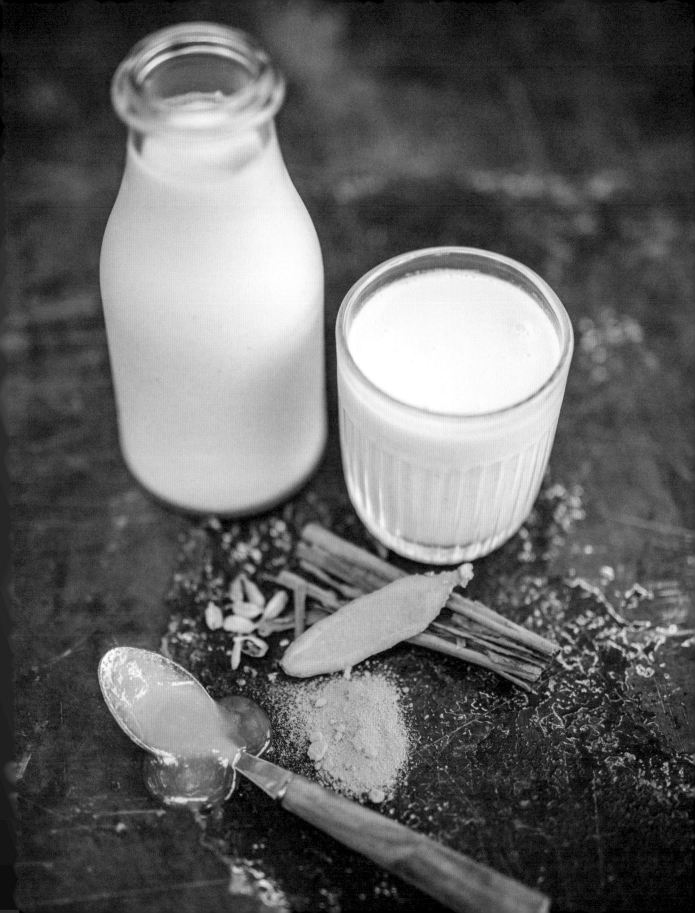

There are endless flavour variations once you figure out your favourite base milk. Try adding fruit and spice to create your own milkshake or protein powders for a superfood shake. Here are some simple suggestions for you to play with. In general, the best rule to follow is one part solids to three parts liquid. Play around with flavours.

BUILD YOUR OWN SHAKE

To build your own shake, choose one ingredient from sections 1 and 2, season with salt at step 3, choose your sweetener at step 4 and then take it in whichever direction you prefer at 5 or 6.

1 Choose your nuts
Almonds, cashews, Brazil nuts, walnuts, pecans, macadamia nuts, hazelnuts, pumpkin seeds, hemp seeds.

2 Spice and flavour
Vanilla powder, cinnamon, cardamom, nutmeg, cacao powder, carob powder.

3 Salt
A pinch of Himalayan salt.

4 Sweetener
Dates, raisins, stevia, raw or manuka honey, maple syrup.

5 Superfood shake
Protein powder of choice, lucuma, maca, activated barley, spirulina, ground flaxseed.

6 Milkshake
Add a handful of your fruit of choice once strained to create a milkshake.

FOR THE BASE MILK:
As on p.141, the general rule is 100g nuts or seeds, soaked for 6 hours, or overnight, to 850ml filtered water.

Blend until smooth and creamy, then strain through a nut milk bag.

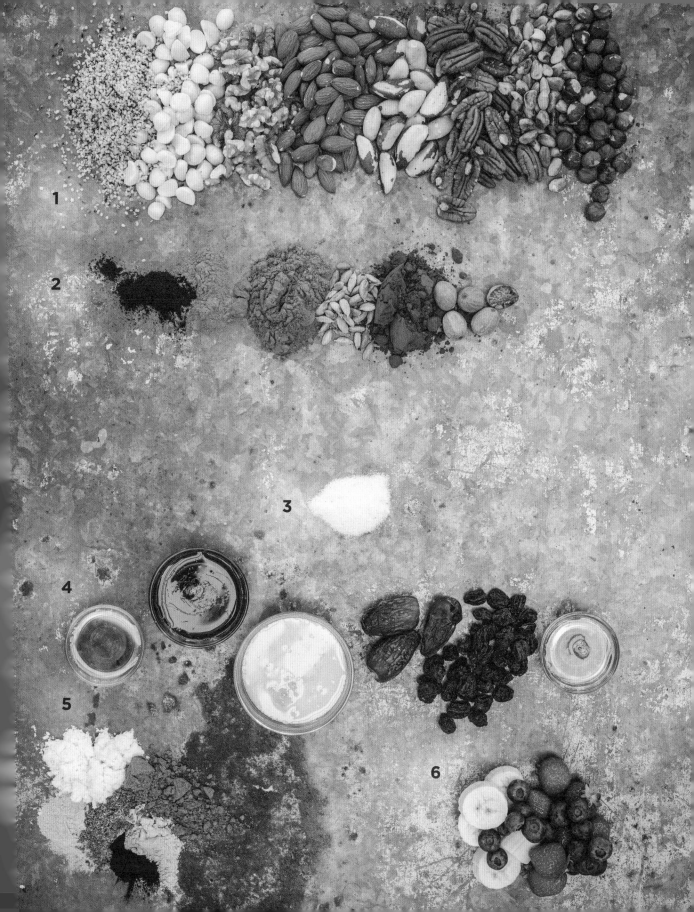

1

2

3

4

5

6

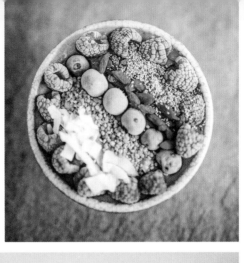

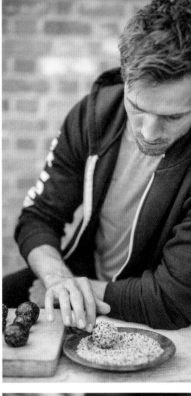

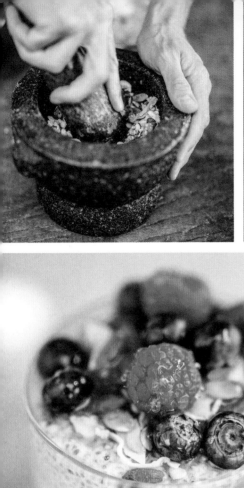

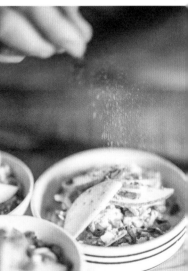

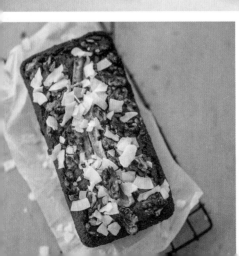

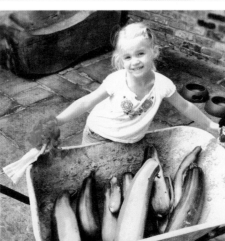

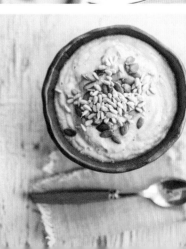

FOOD

BREAKFAST · LIQUID LUNCH
ON THE GO · ICE CREAM

This book is predominantly about liquid, but I love food and wanted to share some of my favourite meals to show how you can integrate them into your life. Your daily consumption should be about how you feel and what you are doing. Listen to your body: if you feel sluggish or that you indulged too much the day/night before, take it easy and have a nice green smoothie for breakfast, salad for lunch and soup for dinner. If you need energy, why not incorporate some high-value foods such as oats, nuts, seeds and green juices.

Here are some of my favourite recipes. If you like them, who knows, I might have to write a Foodman book . . .

BREAKFAST
We all know that breakfast is the most important meal of the day. It is also my favourite meal of the day. Breakfast in my house can easily go on for 3 hours at the weekend!

Eating a good breakfast is a great habit to get into, as you are setting yourself up with all the energy you need to get you through the day. I have included lots of recipes in this section which can be prepared the night before too, for those of us who might not have time in the morning. There really is no excuse to leave the house with an empty tank!

LIQUID LUNCH

Juices and smoothies can be a useful meal replacement or a great way to have a healthy snack on the go. Smoothies are effectively cold soups. This section shows you some more savoury versions, as well as my infamous bone broth. I love soups – they're a staple part of my weekly diet.

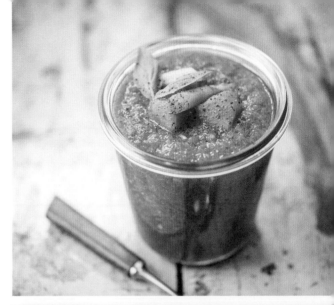

ON THE GO

I'm always on the go – whether I'm flying out of the house at 5am to do some filming or on a road trip with Jane and the kids – so I need snacks! This section is about how to make healthy, easily transportable snacks to take with you wherever you're going. I try to save an evening a week or Sunday morning to make some batches of kale chips and protein balls – and we always have a loaf of Banana Man to hand in my house. Be warned: none of these will last long because they're so delicious, so make a double batch!

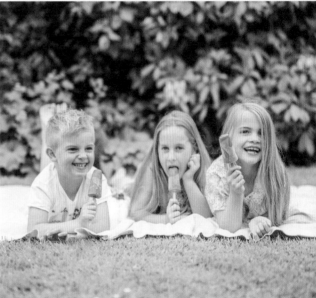

ICE CREAM

I love ice cream – and so does my family. However, my son Jackson has an allergy to dairy. These recipes are all dairy free, guilt free and packed with flavour. Feel free to play around with your favourite fruits and nuts.

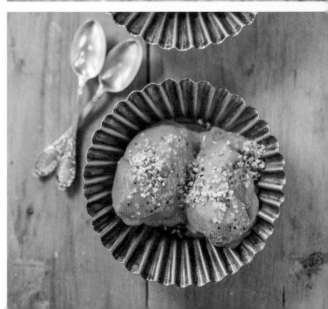

BREAKFAST

MUESLI IN A GLASS

A lovely, quick brekkie in a cup. I use this recipe a lot, as my mornings can be quite hectic. If you don't want gluten, buy gluten-free oats, which can be found in most supermarkets. serves one

2 handfuls of oats, soaked overnight in water and drained	1 apple, cored and chopped
1 Medjool date, pitted	1 tbsp coconut butter
½ tsp ground cinnamon	a handful of ice cubes
1 tbsp almond butter	250ml mineral water or coconut water

Combine all the ingredients in a blender and blitz until smooth.

JUICEMAN TIP
Top this with some pumpkin and sunflower seeds.

CASHEW COFFEE

Coffee and cashews . . . BOOM! This is a fantastic healthy way to enjoy your morning coffee. The cacao will give you an extra kick, too! serves one

half a handful of almonds or cashew nuts, soaked for 6 hours or overnight, drained	1 tsp raw cacao nibs
	1–2 shots of cooled espresso
½ a frozen banana	250ml almond milk
	½ tbsp coconut sugar
	a handful of ice cubes

Combine all the ingredients in a blender and blitz until smooth.

RAW ICED MOCHACHINO

If you usually kick-start your morning with a coffee then you will love my take on a mocha, especially on warm days. It hits all the right spots and gets you ready to conquer the day. serves one

350ml almond milk	1 tbsp coconut butter
1 tsp lucuma powder	1 tbsp raw honey
1 tsp maca powder	6 ice cube
1 tbsp raw cacao powder	

Put all the ingredients into a blender and blitz well until smooth. You can enjoy this drink warm by blending on high for 2 minutes and omitting the ice. Pour the shake into a glass and drink immediately.

JUICEMAN FACT
Lucuma powder is a natural wonder-sweetener packed with vitamins and minerals.

CACAO ESPRESSO

This cacao espresso will give you a definite lift. I have tried this on many of my coffee-loving friends and they have been won over by it as it makes a brilliant coffee substitute. serves one

For the espresso:	a pinch of ground cinnamon
a handful of raw cashew nuts	a pinch of cayenne pepper
225ml mineral water	**For the cashew cream:**
1 tbsp raw cacao nibs	150g cashews
1 tbsp raw cacao powder	3 Medjool dates, pitted
2 tbsp raw honey or agave nectar	250ml water
a pinch of vanilla powder	1 tsp vanilla powder
1 tsp coconut butter	1 tbsp coconut butter

Put all the espresso ingredients into a blender and blitz for at least 1 minute until you have a fairly thick and intense chocolate drink. Feel free to overblend for a hot alternative. Put all the cashew cream ingredients into a blender and blitz until smooth. Pour the cashew cream on top of the espresso for a totally delicious experience.

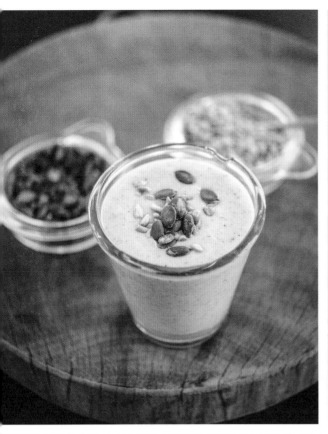

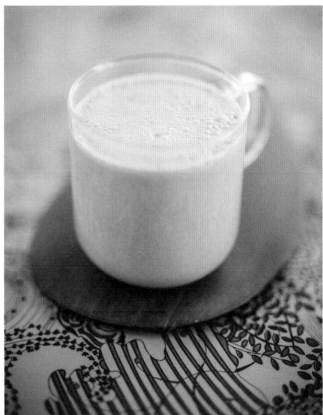

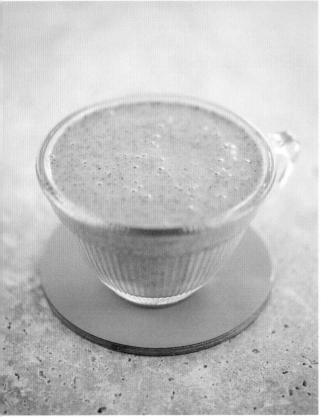

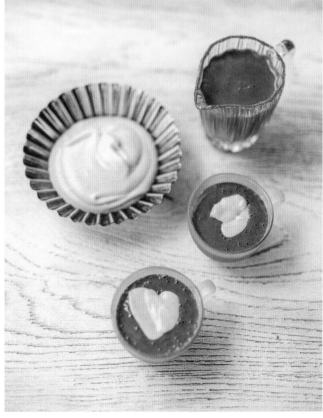

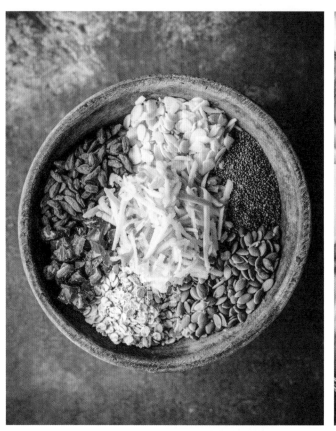

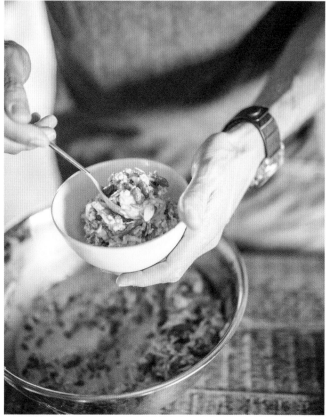

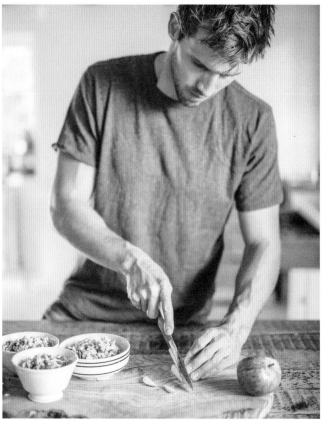

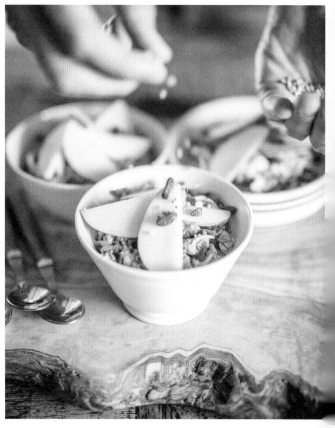

Once you have tried this you will be hooked. It makes breakfast-time easy, fast and nutritious. But don't just save this for breakfast – it is a great snack at any time of day. serves four

OVERNIGHT OATS

300g oats

a handful of flaked almonds

1 apple, cored and grated

a handful of goji berries or raisins

2 tbsp pumpkin seeds

3 tbsp chia seeds

750ml nut milk or coconut milk, plus extra to serve

2 Medjool dates, pitted and chopped

a pinch of ground cinnamon

a pinch of vanilla powder

a pinch of Himalayan salt

a handful of strawberries chopped

maple syrup or raw honey, optional

Place all the ingredients in a bowl except the strawberries and stir until thoroughly mixed. Place in the fridge overnight.

The next morning give the mixture another stir and serve with chopped strawberries and extra nut milk. Add maple syrup or raw honey for added sweetness.

JUICEMAN TIP
Try adding some lucuma powder for extra vitamin B.

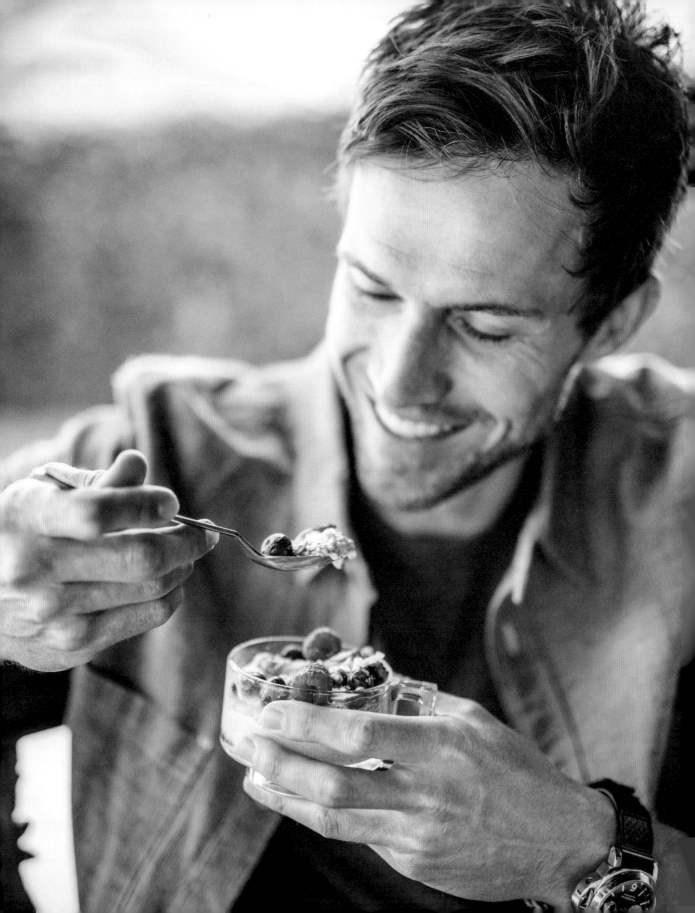

I love chia pots and eat them for breakfast three to four times a week. The basic rule of thumb is one part chia seeds to five parts liquid, which makes a great consistency. Chia seeds are known to give you energy, so this is great to eat at any time of the day. The chia seeds swell in liquid, making them a very filling snack.

makes two small pots

JUICEMAN CHIA POT

250ml almond milk

½ tsp vanilla powder

1 tsp raw honey

4 tbsp chia seeds

Put the almond milk, vanilla and honey into a jug and stir well. Add the chia seeds and keep stirring to make sure they don't stick together. Once mixed well, leave in the fridge for a minimum of 4 hours, or overnight if you have an early start the next day. Top with chopped fruit, berries and pumpkin seeds.

JUICEMAN TIP
Try adding chopped banana, hemp seeds and honey to the bottom of your bowl before you add the chia mixture. It makes it extra delicious and filling.

This is a brilliant example of how versatile juices can be. The carrot and apple juice makes this porridge vitamin-rich and adds sweetness; the coconut butter makes it really creamy. This is a great way to start the day – you will be surprised by how good it tastes. serves two

CARROT AND APPLE PORRIDGE

150g oats

300ml carrot and apple juice (around 3 carrots and 2 apples)

250ml mineral water

1 tsp cinnamon

1 tsp vanilla powder

1–2 tsp coconut butter

your favourite dried fruits and seeds, optional

Place all the ingredients in a pan and warm on a low heat for 8–10 minutes, stirring occasionally to prevent sticking. Add more water depending on your desired consistency. Remove from the heat, transfer to a bowl and top with whatever takes your fancy.

JUICEMAN TIP
I always add the pulp from the juice into the porridge too for extra fibre and goodness.

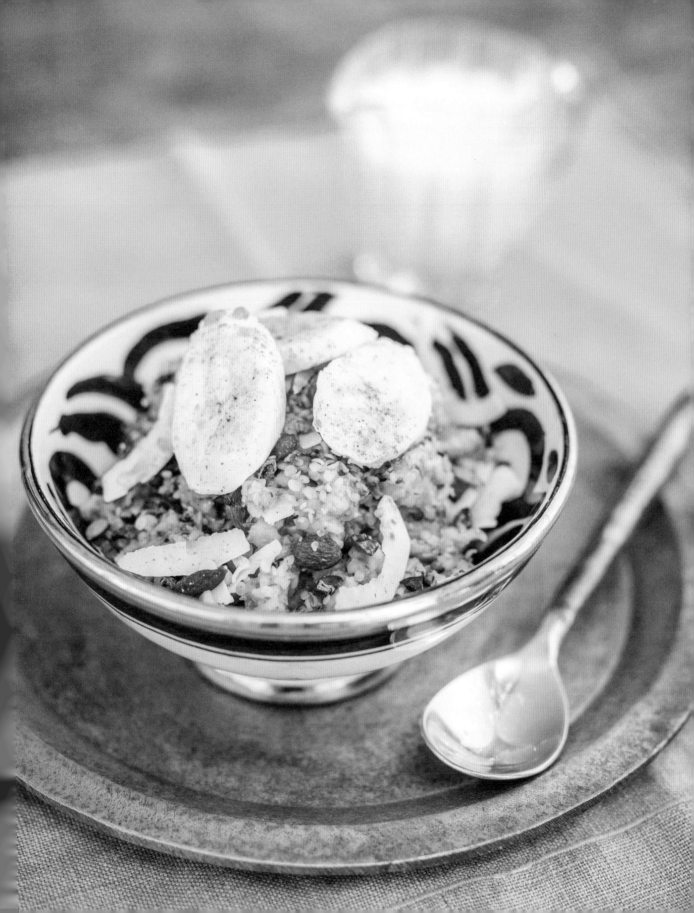

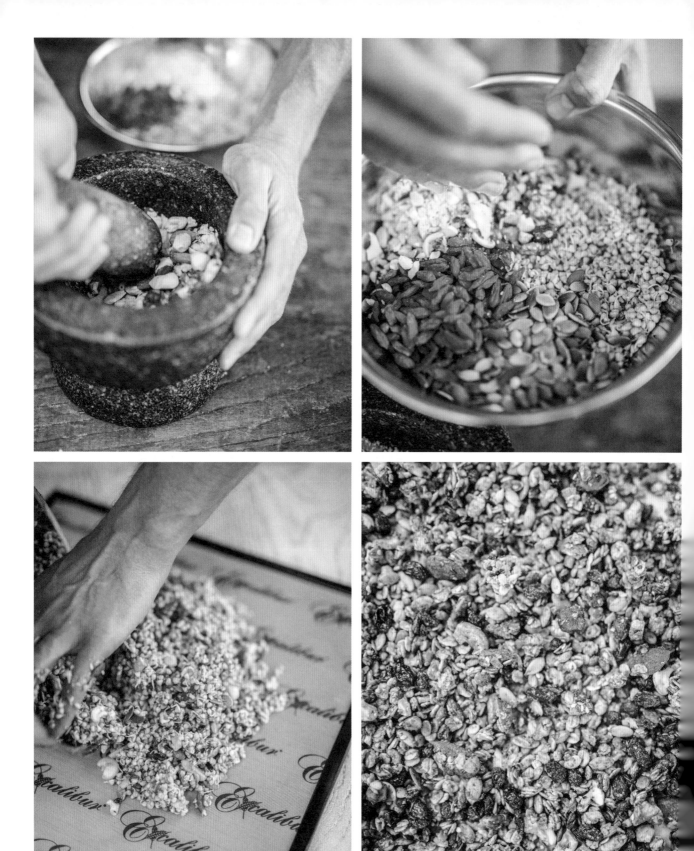

I like to know exactly what ingredients I am eating, so there really isn't anything better than homemade granola – and it is so quick and easy to make. It lasts for ages in an airtight container, too. It can be eaten straight with yogurt or milk. I also like to use it to top a chia pot or to snack on through the day. serves two

EVERYDAY GRANOLA

For the date paste:

5 Medjool dates, pitted

1 tbsp coconut oil

For the granola mix:

200g oats

2 tbsp maple syrup

150g mixed nuts, broken up inside a cloth with a rolling pin

a pinch of vanilla powder

a pinch of ground cinnamon

1 tbsp pumpkin seeds

1 tbsp flaxseeds

Preheat the oven to 180°C/350°F/gas 4. Line a baking tray with parchment paper.

First, make the date paste. Put the dates and the coconut oil in a blender and blitz until smooth.

Combine the date paste with the rest of the granola mix ingredients in a bowl. Spread the mixture out to about 2–4cm thick on the baking tray and place in the pre-heated oven for 30–40 minutes. Check every 10 minutes to make sure it isn't burning and give it a shake.

Once crisp and golden brown, remove from the oven and leave to cool. Store in an airtight container.

GREEN GIANT BREAKFAST BOWL

A smoothie in a bowl is my ultimate breakfast – quick, easy and super-nutritious. Smoothie bowls don't have to be confined to breakfast time though. They can be enjoyed any time of day. serves one

½ an avocado, peeled and destoned	¼ of a chopped frozen pineapple
¼ of a fennel bulb	1 tbsp hemp seeds
a handful of spinach and kale leaves	250ml almond milk or ice-cold mineral water
1cm piece of fresh root ginger, peeled	a handful of ice cubes
1 frozen banana	

Place all the ingredients into a blender and blitz until smooth. Pour into a bowl and top with seeds, nuts or granola (p.161).

EXOTIC SMOOTHIE BOWL

Once you start making morning smoothie bowls you'll never stop. This version works really well and is packed with nutrition. Unless I am training in the gym, this will easily see me through till my next meal. The consistency should be thick like ice cream so you will need a spoon or spatula to get it out. serves one

1 frozen banana	1 tbsp chia seeds
1 mango, peeled and chopped	1 tbsp natural protein powder
¼ tsp turmeric powder	a handful of frozen blueberries
115g coconut yogurt or kefir	a handful of fresh strawberries

Place all the ingredients in a blender and blitz to a thick consistency. Top with granola, fresh fruit and seeds – ready to eat and become your new obsession!

BLUEBERRY, COCONUT & CHIA SMOOTHIE BOWL

serves one

60ml coconut water	1 tbsp coconut butter or coconut oil
a handful of frozen blueberries	1 tsp goji berries
1 frozen banana	1 tsp chia seeds
	1 tbsp natural protein powder

Place all the ingredients in a blender and blitz to a thick consistency. Pour into a bowl and sprinkle on the toppings of your choice.

FOREVER YOUNG SMOOTHIE BOWL

Matcha tea is the best-quality powdered green tea available. It contains five times as many antioxidants as other foods, which are the magical nutrients and enzymes responsible for fighting UV damage, giving us younger-looking skin. serves one

180ml mineral water	1 tsp matcha green tea powder
a handful of baby spinach leaves	1 frozen banana
½ an avocado, peeled and destoned	2 handfuls of chopped frozen pineapple
1 lime, peeled	a handful of ice cubes
1 tbsp coconut butter	
1 tbsp raw honey	

Place all the ingredients in a blender and blitz until smooth. Adjust the sweetness if desired by adding more honey or a date. Pour into a bowl and sprinkle on the toppings of your choice.

JUICEMAN TIP
Top with blueberries, raw cacao and goji berries for an antioxidant feast. See the photo for inspiration.

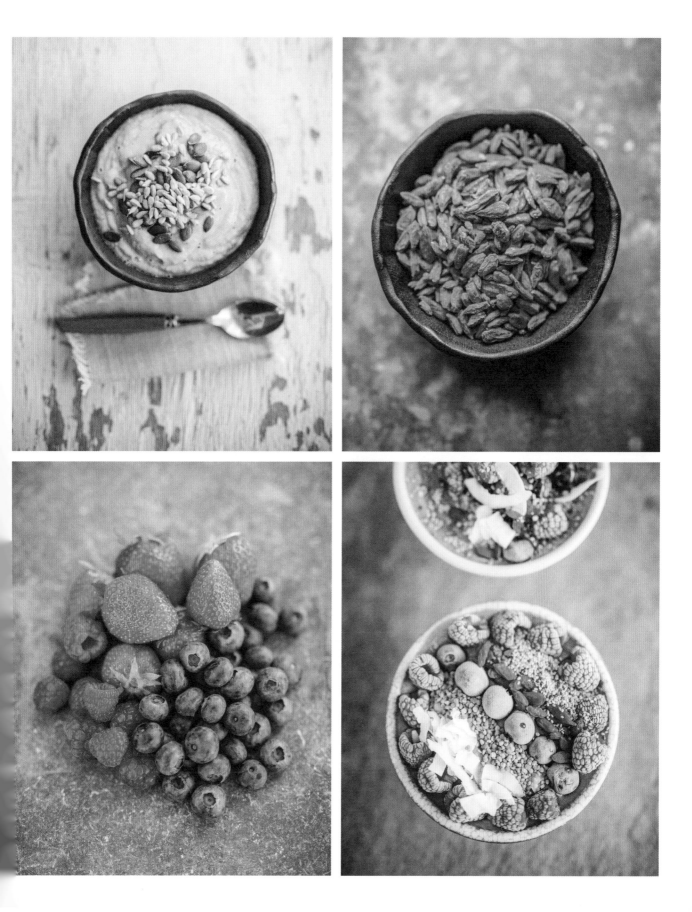

LIQUID LUNCH

This was something that I only started making last year as a result of a very serious gut infection which I picked up on my travels. At one point I was diagnosed with Crohn's disease, which led me to search for the best things to heal my stomach and gut. The diagnosis was unbelievably scary but luckily I'm now in remission, helped along by plenty of rest and this medicinal soup. It's packed with amino acids, collagen, glucosamine, silicon, magnesium and many other nutrients besides. Making this broth is now a weekly ritual for me. On Sundays we always roast a chicken and make this broth with the bones. You will be amazed by how easy it is, as well as by the amount of food you can make from one chicken!

BONE BROTH

1.6kg chicken, preferably organic

Himalayan salt and black pepper

1 tbsp coconut oil

2 onions, peeled and roughly chopped

3 celery sticks roughly chopped

4 carrots, roughly chopped

3 bay leaves

2 sprigs of rosemary

a glug of apple cider vinegar

200g brown rice or kelp noodles (optional)

Pre-heat the oven to 180°C/350°F/gas 4.

Place your bird in a large casserole pot and season well with the salt, pepper and coconut oil. I use the back of a spoon to spread the oil evenly over the chicken.

Roast for 1 hour and then add 500ml of water and return the pot to the oven for a further 30 minutes.

Remove the chicken and allow to cool. Take off all the meat from the bones and set aside.

Place the chicken carcass back into the pot, along with the vegetables, herbs, vinegar and 2 litres of water. Cook in the oven for a minimum of 4 hours at 120°C/250°F/gas ½.

Strain the liquid into a separate saucepan. Add half the chicken meat (you can use the rest of the meat in your favourite salad or wrap) and brown rice or kelp noodles. Place back in the oven for 20 minutes.

Remove the saucepan from the oven. Now is the time to add in whatever fresh ingredients and flavours take your fancy. Here are some ideas which have worked for me:

Fresh veg: kale, sliced carrots, pak choi, mushrooms, beansprouts, peppers.

Spices: grated fresh ginger or turmeric, sliced fresh chilli, roast garlic puree.

Fresh herbs: parsley, chives, coriander.

JUICEMAN TIP
You can freeze the broth for later use. We always have frozen broth on hand to use in soups and gravy or to even drink straight up.

JUICEMAN FACT
Bone broth is easy for our bodies to absorb and contains minerals such as calcium, silicon, sulphur, magnesium, phosphorous and many trace minerals.

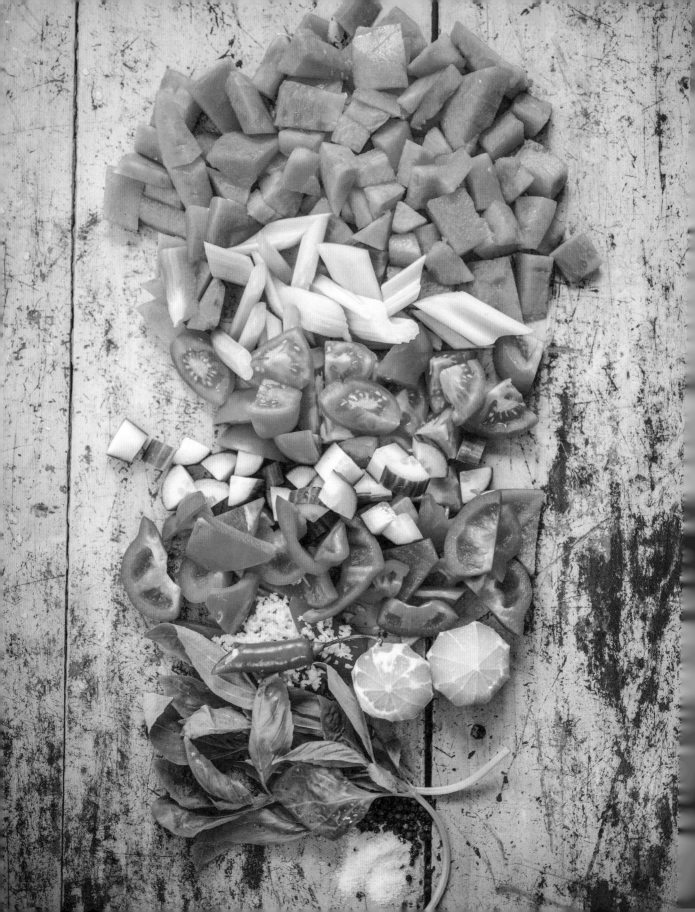

I love gazpacho – this is a bit of a different take on it, but it works really nicely. The ginger and the chilli give it a bit of a kick, but you can put in as little or as much as you like. It can be served in bowls or glasses. serves two

WATERMELON GAZPACHO

½ a watermelon, peeled, seeded and chopped into 2.5cm cubes

2 celery sticks, chopped

3 medium tomatoes, roughly chopped

½ a cucumber, roughly chopped

2 red bell peppers, roughly chopped

2.5cm piece of fresh root ginger, peeled and minced

½ a red chilli

the juice of 2 limes

a handful of fresh basil leaves

Himalayan salt and black pepper

1 tbsp apple cider vinegar

Put 2 or 3 cubes of the watermelon and a couple of celery pieces into your bowls or glasses. Pour the remaining ingredients into a blender. Pulse until it reaches a soup-like consistency. Taste it and add more seasoning if needed. Chill in the fridge for 2–3 hours before serving.

JUICEMAN TIP
Traditionally, the Spanish add bread to their gazpacho, which gives it a creamy texture. Try adding a handful of soaked cashew nuts to this recipe for the same effect.

There is a fine line between a smoothie and a soup. I would call this a savoury smoothie or chilled soup, so you can choose how you want to eat it. Either way, it's delicious. Go easy with the spice at first – you can always blend and then add more to taste. *serves two*

SPICY AVOCADO AND CARROT SOUP

the juice of 6 carrots

1 large avocado, peeled

1½ tbsp grated fresh root ginger

1½ tbsp lemon juice

½ a green chilli

¼ tsp cayenne pepper

a small bunch of mint

a small bunch of basil

2 tbsp cold-pressed olive oil

Put the carrot juice into a blender with the rest of the ingredients and blitz to your desired consistency. I like it smooth. Drizzle with a little olive oil and sprinkle with cayenne pepper before serving.

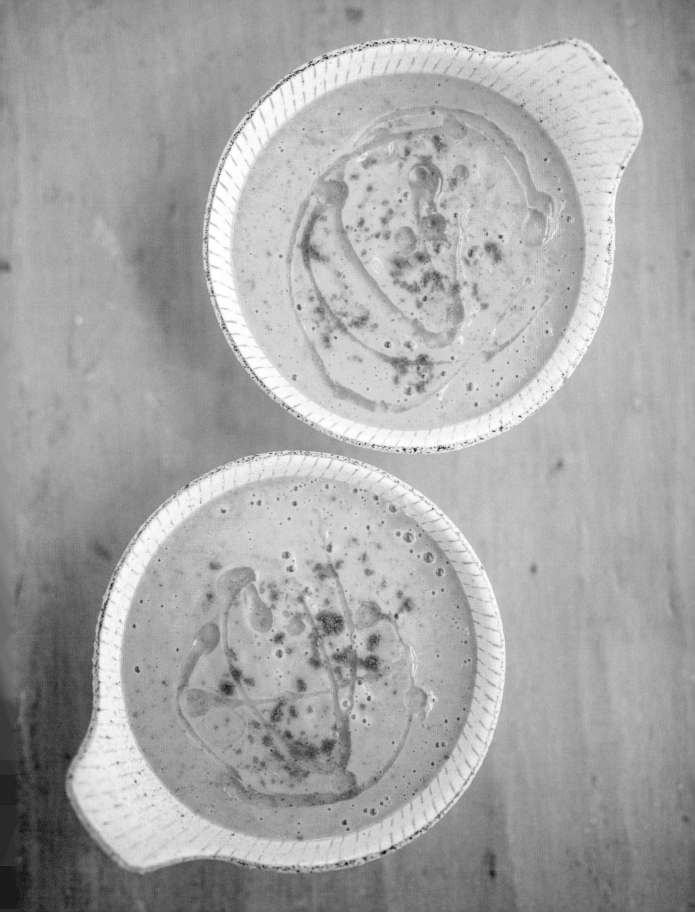

Everyone loves a banana cake, and this dairy- and wheat-free version is amazing. My kids love a slice with a thick helping of raw honey spread on top. Nut butter works well too.
makes one loaf cake

BANANA MAN

300g ripe bananas

3 eggs

2 tbsp chia seeds

150g ground almonds

50g ground flaxseeds

1 tbsp hemp protein

3 tbsp raw honey

2 tsp cold-pressed hemp oil

1 tbsp cold-pressed olive oil

1 tsp ground cinnamon

1 tsp coconut butter

2 tsp bicarbonate of soda

the juice of 1 lemon

a pinch of Himalayan salt

Optional toppings:

sliced banana

walnuts

coconut flakes

Preheat the oven to 180°C/350°F/gas 4.

Place the ingredients in a blender in the order listed. Blend until the mixture is smooth and then set aside for 10 minutes.

In the meantime, grease a medium-size loaf tin and line it with flaxseeds or extra chia seeds which will help prevent the mixture from sticking. Pour in the mix and give it a gentle shake to level the surface. Top with sliced banana and walnuts.

Bake in the oven for 30 minutes. Keep checking it and put tin foil over the top if it starts to burn.

The centre needs to be firm so check with a knife and if it comes out clean it's done.

Sprinkle with coconut flakes before serving, if you like.

JUICEMAN TIP
Try adding maca powder to the mixture for extra power.

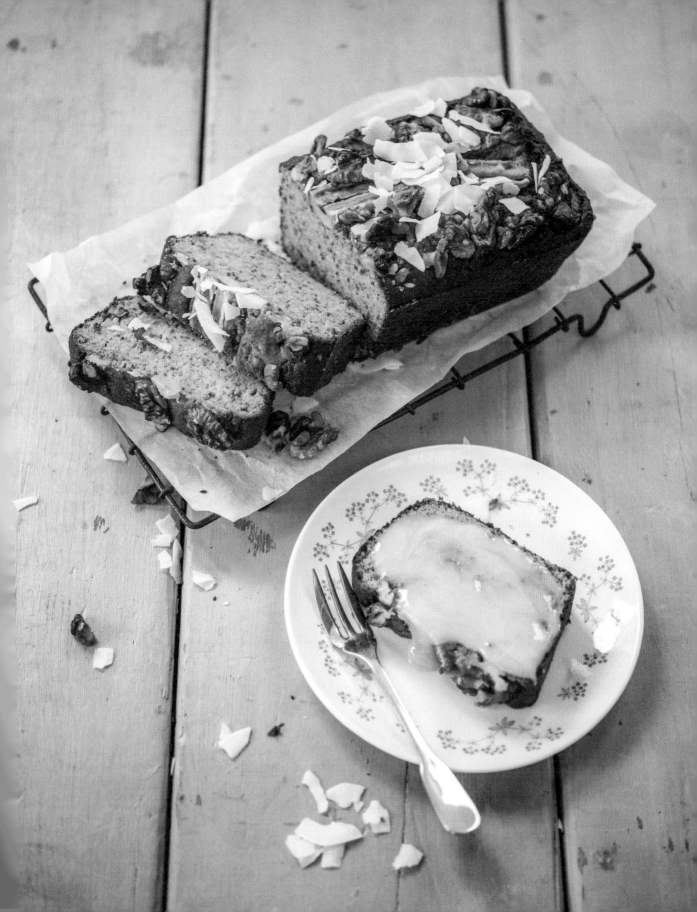

These protein balls are great for snacking on and for eating after training. They are absolutely delicious and look spectacular – even my kids love them! I make a batch on Sunday for the week ahead. *makes 25 truffles*

JUICEMAN PROTEIN TRUFFLES

For the truffles:

150g almonds

150g cashew nuts

100g pumpkin seeds

½ tsp sea salt

½ tsp ground cinnamon

1 tbsp chocolate protein or hemp protein powder

1 tbsp maca powder

1 tbsp raw cacao nibs

2 tsp spirulina powder

18 Medjool dates, pitted

a squeeze of orange or lemon juice

1 tbsp coconut oil

For the toppings:

1 tbsp raw cacao powder

1 tbsp hemp seeds

a handful of goji berries, chopped

1 tbsp grated coconut

Put all the ingredients for the truffles into a blender and pulse until it forms a thick, smooth consistency. Then roll the mixture into small balls. To finish, roll the balls in the cacao powder, hemp seeds, goji berries or grated coconut. Sometimes I mix the toppings together and cover the truffles in all of them.

JUICEMAN TIP
For a bit of variation in flavour, try adding lemon zest and a pinch of vanilla powder to the truffle mixture, or some orange zest and finely chopped chilli.

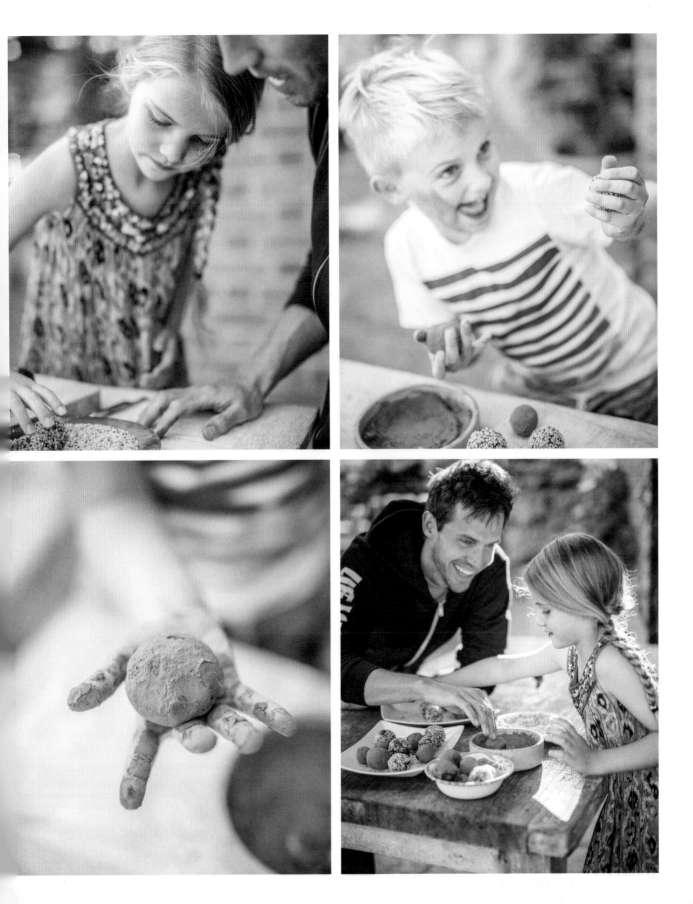

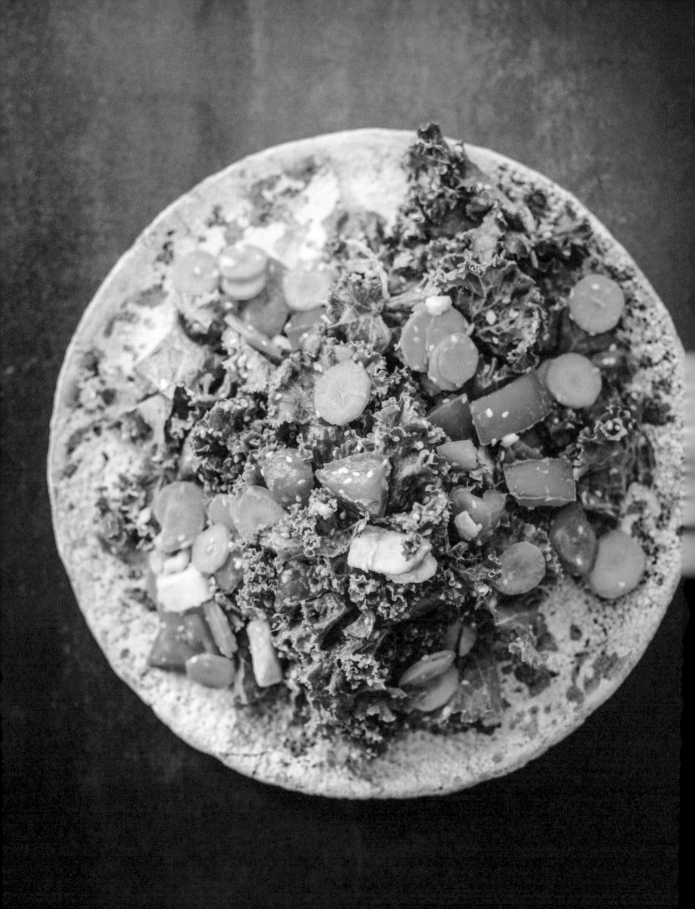

Ever since I started Juiceman I have been making salads made with juice ingredients and vice versa. Kale is such a powerhouse of nutrients and when it's massaged with lemon, oil and salt it becomes a great base for lots of different salad variations – from kale chicken caesar to kale waldorf. The key is to fully coat the kale leaves with the dressing and massage well. Unlike other salads, this one will also keep overnight because of its dense texture.

serves two

Option 1

a handful of alfalfa sprouts

1 tbsp pumpkin seeds

2 tbsp pomegranate seeds

Option 2

a handful of raisins

1 celery stick, sliced

1 head of chicory, roughly chopped

Option 3

2 handfuls of black olives

1 red onion, sliced

½ a cucumber, chopped

Option 4

2 tomatoes, chopped

a handful of rocket

1 mozzarella ball, sliced

KALE SALAD

2 large handfuls of kale (approx. 6 large leaves)

a pinch of Himalayan salt

2 carrots

1 lemon

½–1 avocado, peeled, and roughly chopped

2 large tomatoes, chopped

1 tbsp sesame seeds

For the dressing:

3 tbsp cold-pressed olive oil

the juice of ½ a lemon

1 tsp hemp oil

1 tbsp apple cider vinegar

1 tsp honey

Himalayan salt and black pepper

Remove the stalks from the kale, wash and rip or chop. Place in a large bowl. Sprinkle the kale with salt and massage into the leaves. Leave for 5 minutes to soften.

Meanwhile, peel your carrots and slice as thin as possible. A mandolin does the job perfectly.

Squeeze the lemon over the kale, add the avocado and mix thoroughly. Add the carrots, tomatoes and sesame seeds and season to your liking.

Mix the ingredients for the dressing together and drizzle over the salad.

Why not try the combinations at the top of the page too, either instead of the tomatoes and carrots or as extra toppings.

I am such a fan of kale chips. They can be coated in all sorts of flavours, from maple and cinnamon to honey, but this spicy citrus recipe is my favourite. The amounts I've given will make 3–4 trays full, but it's better to make a big batch as they can be stored easily in an airtight container. However, they are so delicious that they generally get hoovered up pretty quickly in our house!

JUICEMAN'S KILLER KALE CHIPS

10 kale leaves

1 tsp Himalayan salt

1 tbsp cold-pressed olive oil or coconut oil

the juice of 1 lemon

1 tbsp nutritional yeast

1 tbsp chilli powder or a red chilli

1 tbsp ground cumin powder

1 tbsp smoked paprika

150g cashew nuts

½ tsp cayenne pepper

Preheat your oven to 150°C/300°F/gas 2. Line a large baking sheet with parchment paper or, if using a dehydrator, place sheets on your dehydrator trays.

Wash the kale well then remove and discard the stalks. Roughly tear the leaves up, add them to a bowl with the salt and scrunch well.

Throw the remaining ingredients into a blender and blitz until smooth. Add this mixture to the bowl with the kale leaves and toss until fully coated.

Spread out the kale leaves on the prepared baking sheet and place in the oven for 20 minutes, turning halfway through. If using a dehydrator, select 125°F–145°F for 6 hours, turning halfway through.

Remove and leave to cool down and crisp up before enjoying.

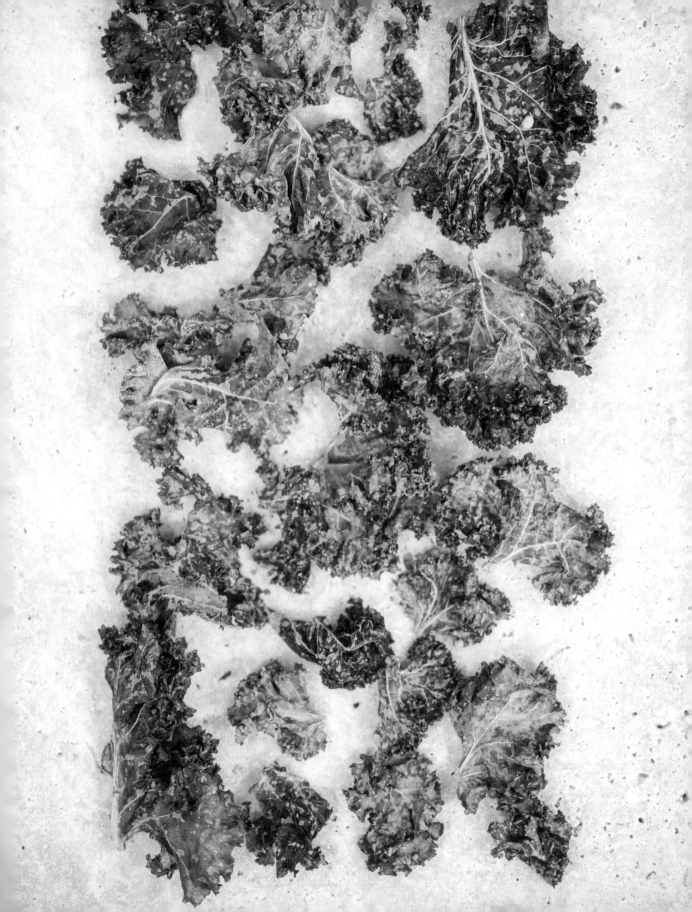

ICE CREAM

ALMOND STRAWBERRY ICE CREAM

In the summer months I freeze lots of organic strawberries so that I can make this at any time of year. serves two

4 handfuls of frozen strawberries	1 tbsp maple syrup (optional)
250ml almond milk	hemp seeds (optional)
1 tbsp almond butter or coconut butter	

Place all the ingredients in your blender and blitz until smooth. Use your tamper if you have one to get a smooth texture. Do not overblend so that the mixture gets hot. Transfer the mixture to a tub and freeze, or enjoy straight away sprinkled with hemp seeds and a drizzle of maple syrup.

BANANA & CASHEW ICE CREAM

My kids call this vanilla ice cream . . . Little do they know! This is another great way to use your stash of frozen bananas. serves two

2 frozen bananas	a pinch of vanilla powder
250ml cashew milk	1 tbsp raw honey, plus extra for drizzling
1 tbsp nut butter or coconut butter	

Place all the ingredients in your blender and blitz until smooth. Use your tamper if you have one to get a smooth texture. Do not overblend so that the mixture gets hot. Transfer the mixture to a tub and freeze, or enjoy straight with an extra drizzle of honey.

VANILLA CACAO ICE CREAM

For ice cream or smoothies it is always a good idea to have frozen nut milk on hand. I use a simple ice cube tray. Once the milk is frozen, you can transfer the ice cubes to a zip lock bag and keep them for up to three months in the freezer. Play with the amount of liquid per cube, depending on what size cube your blender can cope with. serves two

1 frozen banana	1 tbsp raw cacao nibs, plus extra for serving
6 nut milk ice cubes, or 225ml nut milk	1 tsp raw cacao powder
a pinch of vanilla powder	1 tbsp maple syrup

Place all the ingredients in your blender and blitz until smooth. Use your tamper if you have one to get a smooth texture. Do not overblend so that the mixture gets hot. Transfer the mixture to a tub and freeze, or enjoy straight away with sprinkled with extra cacao nibs.

MANGO SORBET

Sorbet in its simplest form is my favourite dessert on a hot day. You can use any fruit to make this recipe. My daughter loves it with frozen raspberries, but I think it works best with mango. serves two

1½ frozen mangoes	1 lime or ½ an orange, peeled

Place all the ingredients in your blender and blitz until smooth. Use your tamper if you have one to get a smooth texture. Do not overblend so that the mixture gets hot. Transfer the mixture to a tub and freeze, or enjoy straight away.

JUICEMAN TIP
Try mixing in some frozen chopped peaches for a change. I also like to add some freshly chopped mint leaves to complement the mango, or some chilli for a spicy version.

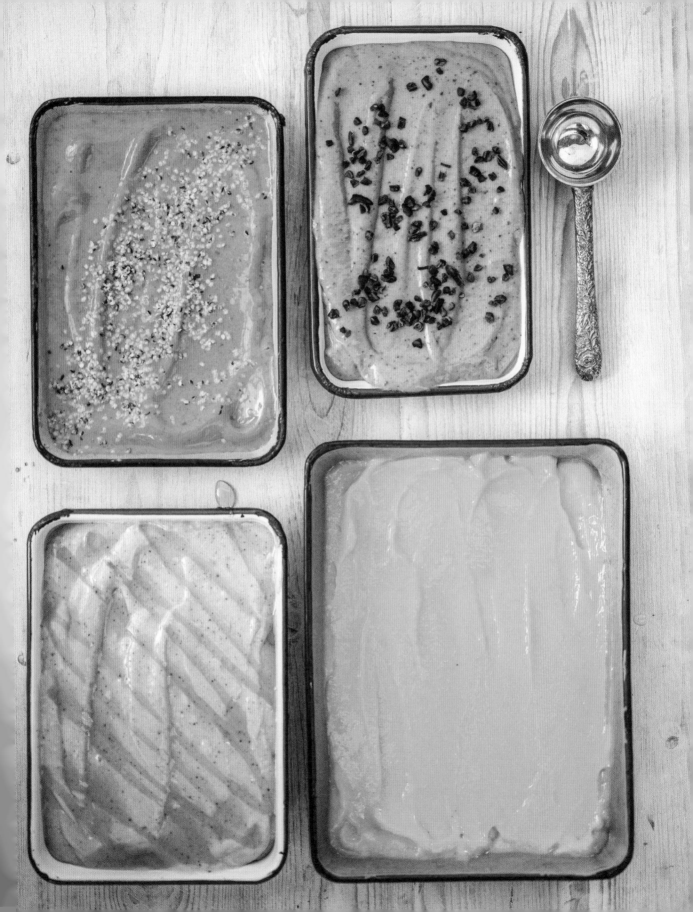

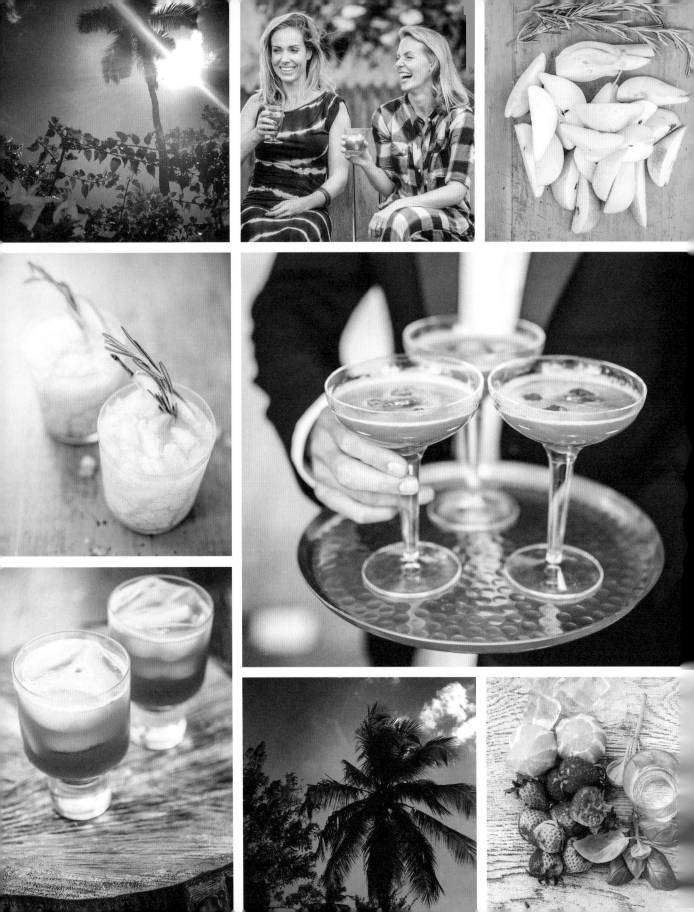

COCKTAILS

Juicing can also provide some fun – in a guilt-free way of course! Cold-pressed cocktails are my passion and my Friday night ritual. So much so, that I'm now partnering up with a huge spirits company, as they were fed up with serving their premium drinks with sodas – I can totally see why. What better way to enjoy your cocktail than with a healthy fresh mixer?

As I explained in the main introduction, throughout the book you will also see the cocktail logo next to certain juices that work well with alcohol. Realistically, you can mix your poison with any of your favourite juices, no matter what they are.

You really can have healthy cocktails and they taste better than any pre-boiled, sugar-based drinks served in fancy bars and costing the earth.

My advice for this section is to buy the best-quality alcohol you can afford. My favourite spirits to make cocktails with are vodka, gin, tequila and sake – all of which I call 'clean' spirits. This means they are highly distilled and low in sugar.

And, of course, remember to drink responsibly!

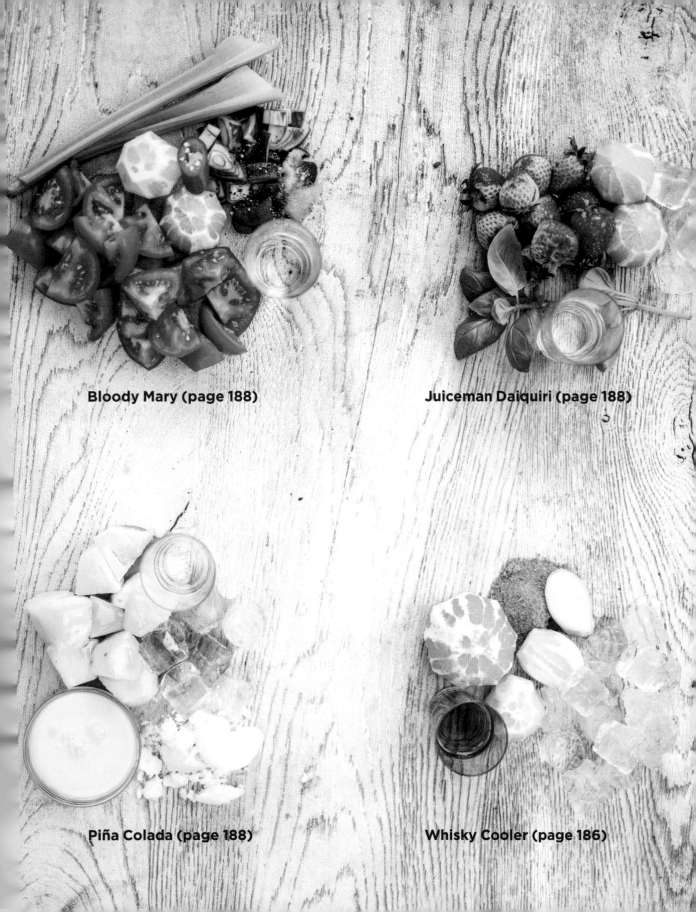

Bloody Mary (page 188)

Juiceman Daiquiri (page 188)

Piña Colada (page 188)

Whisky Cooler (page 186)

RED HOT

I can drink this cocktail all night – it's delicious, with or without the vodka.

serves two

2 handfuls of raspberries

¼ of a red chilli

1 lime, peeled

1 apple

vodka (choose your measure)

Juice all the ingredients and then add as much vodka as you like.

JUICEMAN TIP
This one looks great in a martini glass, served with a couple of raspberries. Grate a little of the lime zest over the top for added zing.

WATERMELON MARTINI

Perfect for a summer party, this cocktail is an all-round people-pleaser. Make sure you have lots of watermelon on tap, as it will all be gone before you know it.

serves two

a handful of strawberries

¼ of a watermelon

a small bunch of mint

1 lime, peeled

vodka (choose your measure)

Juice all the ingredients and then add as much vodka as you want.

JUICEMAN TIP
Try swapping the mint for red chilli for a spicy alternative.

COCONUT WONDER

This reminds me of the many happy holidays I've had in the Caribbean. There is always a good excuse to drink rum, and this is definitely one of them. This drink is refreshing as well as hydrating – forgetting the rum, of course! serves two

½ a pineapple, peeled and cored

1 lime, peeled

250ml coconut water

rum (choose your measure)

Juice the pineapple and lime, then add the coconut water and as much rum as you want.

BROOKLYN BANGER

Whisky is my drink. I personally like it neat with lemon and cloves, but this is a way to make it into a gorgeous long drink to sip all evening. serves two

1 orange, peeled

1 grapefruit, peeled

2.5cm piece of fresh root ginger, peeled

a pinch of cayenne pepper

100ml mineral water

whisky (choose your measure)

Juice the orange, grapefruit and ginger, then add the cayenne pepper, water and as much whisky as you like. Serve over ice.

This is a great way to show how you can adapt simple juices into mixers. Try this citrus cooler with a twist. serves two

WHISKY COOLER

2 lemons, peeled

1 orange, peeled

2.5cm piece of fresh root ginger, peeled

2 tbsp coconut sugar

150ml bourbon

Juice the lemons, orange and ginger. Add the coconut sugar and bourbon and serve over ice with a twist of orange peel.

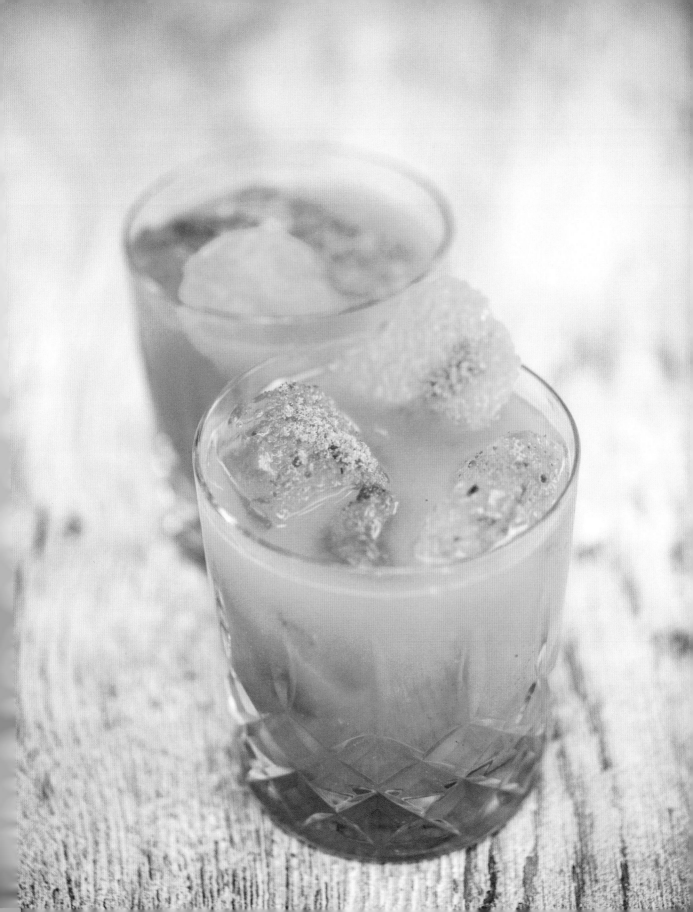

PIÑA COLADA

This fresh take on a piña colada is show-stopping. It's delicious and moreish, so be careful how much rum you use! serves two

1 tbsp coconut butter	250ml coconut milk or mineral water
1 tsp coconut oil	a handful of ice cubes
1 tsp maple syrup	white rum (choose your measure)
a large handful of chopped frozen pineapple	

Place all the ingredients into a blender and blitz until smooth. Serve over ice.

JUICEMAN SANGRIA

I have made this at many family parties and it has always gone down a storm. I love Pinot Noir, and this is an amazing way to drink it. Keep the jug topped up with lots of ice and slices of fresh orange and apple. makes one large jug

½ a pineapple, peeled and cored	a pinch of ground cinnamon
2 pears	1 orange, peeled and sliced
1 lime, peeled	1 apple, sliced
2.5cm piece of fresh root ginger, peeled	a handful of mint leaves
1 bottle of Pinot Noir	a handful of ice cubes
a pinch of vanilla powder	

Juice the pineapple, pears, lime and ginger. In the meantime, pour the Pinot Noir into a jug, add the remaining ingredients to the jug and stir well. Then add the juice, and keep chilled. I love to add loads of different fruit, and it's also great if you replace the Pinot Noir with sparkling wine or champagne.

JUICEMAN TIPS
You can add some agave syrup or coconut sugar for some sweetness. This one works well with flavoured ice cubes (see picture opposite).

BLOODY MARY

I have tried a Bloody Mary in virtually every country I have visited. Some have been great and some not so great. This one, however, is sensational. My wife doesn't usally drink Bloody Marys but is hooked on this one. If you don't believe me, try it! serves two

3 large tomatoes, chopped	1 tbsp tomato purée
2 celery sticks, chopped	60ml vodka
1 lemon, peeled	grated fresh horseradish, to taste, or a pinch of cayenne pepper for extra spice
1 lime, peeled	
½ a red onion, chopped	salt and black pepper, to taste
1 slice of red chilli	

Place all the ingredients, apart from the salt and pepper, in a blender and blitz for 1 minute. If you like it smooth you can press the mixture through a fine sieve using a spoon. Season to taste, and if you want to add some naughty Worcestershire sauce and Tabasco, go for it!

JUICEMAN TIP
Watermelons and tomatoes are a match made in heaven. Try adding some chopped watermelon for a sweeter version in the summer heat.

JUICEMAN DAIQUIRI

We all love a daiquiri, and using fresh ingredients is a must to make this drink banging. Its vibrant colour is not the only reason to drink it. serves two

60ml rum	2 limes, peeled
2 handfuls of frozen strawberries	1 tbsp agave syrup
3 basil leaves	a handful of ice cubes

Place all the ingredients in a blender and blitz until smooth.

JUICEMAN TIP
Add some chopped red chilli for an extra kick.

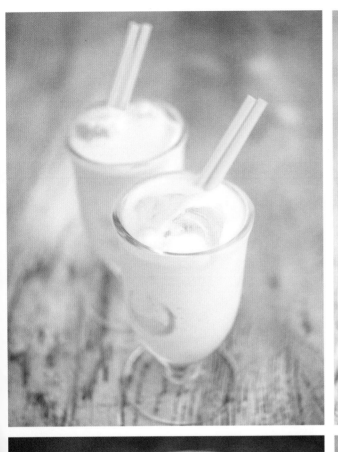

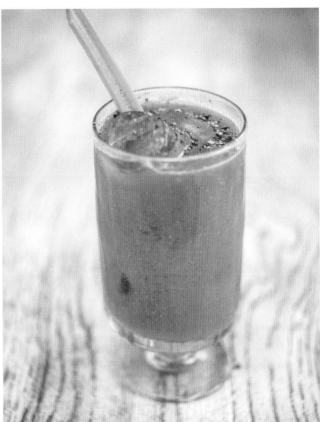

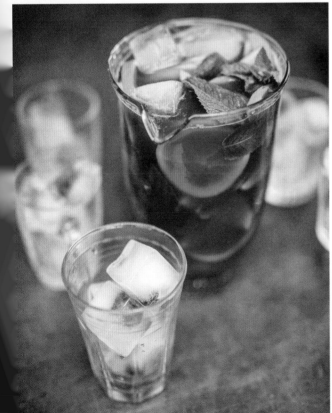

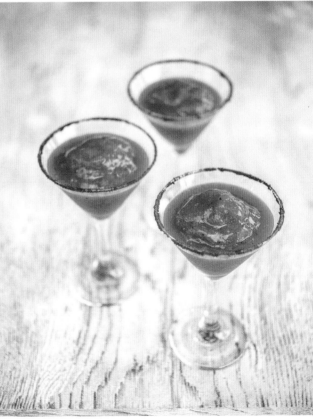

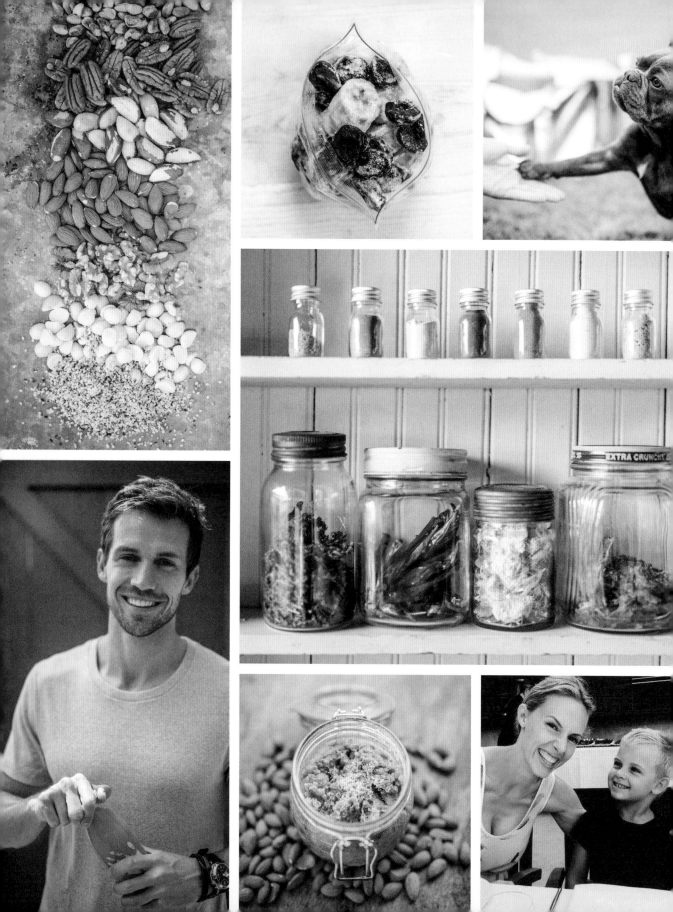

WASTE
NOT
WANT
NOT

When I first started Juiceman.co, one of the things that really interested me was finding ways to use our leftover pulp. I wanted the company to have a zero waste policy and to use our waste product, instead of throwing it away. We have tried everything from teas to dog treats in an attempt to make a company that loves the environment as much as it loves making juices. I wanted to share some easy ways to use your leftovers here, too.

As well as the recipes in this chapter, try adding fruit and veg pulp to cake recipes, porridge and breads. The pulp contains lots of nutrients and of course it's full of fibre, which is great for our digestive systems.

GREEN JUICE PULP CRACKERS

100g green juice pulp
(the greener the better)

2 tbsp ground flaxseeds

1 tbsp tamari or low-sodium soy sauce

2 tbsp nutritional yeast

the juice of 1 lemon

200ml mineral water

2 tbsp chia seeds

Place the pulp, flaxseeds, tamari, nutritional yeast and lemon juice in a blender or food processor. Add the water while blending to get a paste. Transfer to a bowl, add the chia seeds and mix thoroughly.

In the oven:
Preheat the oven to 150°C/300°F/gas 2. Line a large, rimmed baking sheet with parchment paper. Spread the mixture out on the tray and score into 2-inch squares. Cook for 45 minutes, checking regularly.

MY BROTHER MARK'S PULP CRACKERS

100g pulp

2 tbsp ground flaxseeds

2 tbsp tamari or low-sodium soya sauce

2 tsp ground coriander

the juice of ½ a lime

a pinch of Himalayan salt and black pepper

200ml mineral water

2 tbsp chia seeds

Place the pulp, flaxseeds, tamari, coriander, lime and salt and black pepper in a blender or food processor. Add the water while blending to get a paste. Transfer to a bowl, add the chia seeds and mix thoroughly.

In a dehydrator:
Spread the mixture out on a Teflex sheet, score into 2-inch squares and dehydrate at 120°F for 5–6 hours. Flip the sheet over (you may want to put another sheet on top and then flip them both), then dehydrate for a further 4–5 hours until very dry.

My favourite use for leftover pulp is to make wheat-free crackers. My brother Mark is wheat intolerant, so I first made them for him. They were an instant hit. They work well with homemade houmous or as an accompaniment to bone broth or other soups – or simply enjoy them on their own. They are full of flavour, fibre and vital nutrients.

JUICEMAN PULP CRACKERS

100g pulp

3 tbsp ground flaxseeds

2 tbsp chia seeds

2 tbsp sunflower seeds or pumpkin seeds

1 tsp Himalayan salt

1 tsp ground cumin

1 tsp paprika

a pinch of cayenne

the juice of ½ a lime

200ml mineral water

Place all the ingredients in a blender or food processor. Add the water while blending to get a paste.

In the oven:
Preheat the oven to 150°C/300°F/gas 2. Line a large, rimmed baking sheet with parchment paper. Spread the mixture out on the tray and score into 2-inch squares. Cook for 45 minutes, checking regularly.

In a dehydrator:
Spread the mixture out on a Teflex sheet, score into 2-inch squares and dehydrate at 120°F for 5–6 hours. Flip the sheet over (you may want to put another sheet on top and then flip them both), then dehydrate for a further 4–5 hours until very dry.

JUICEMAN TIP
Add a tablespoon of psyllium husk for added fibre. If your mixture gets too thick, add some water or juice.

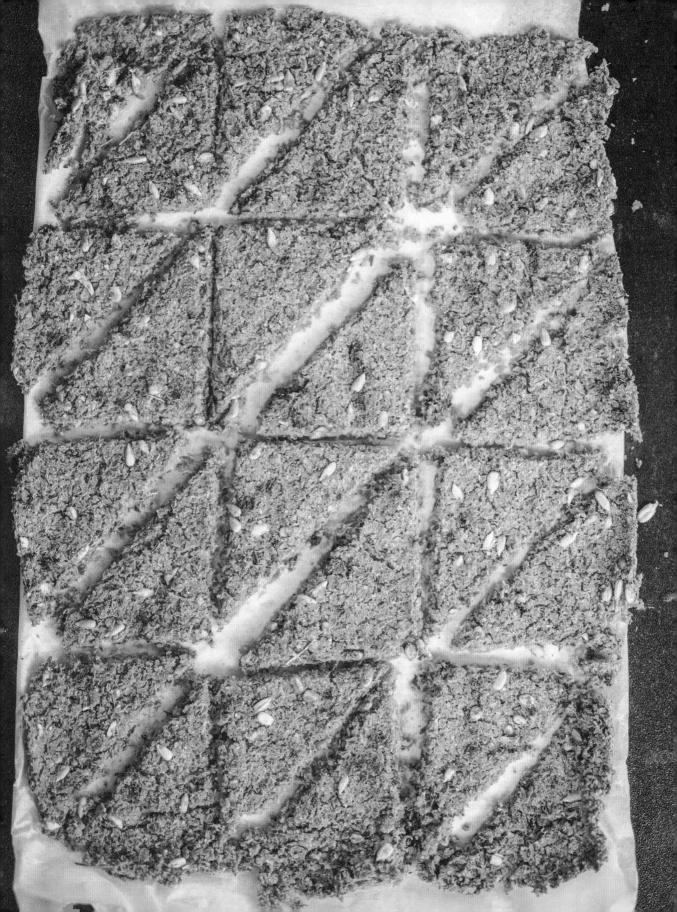

ALMOND PULP BODY SCRUB

This is another brilliant way to use up leftover nut pulp. Any nut pulp will work. My wife used this scrub when she was pregnant to keep good circulation and her skin moisturized. She added wheat germ oil, carrot seed oil and neroli oil. She swears the scrub was the reason she didn't get stretch marks.

50g almond pulp

1 tbsp finely ground sea or crystal salt

1 tsp ground black pepper

1 tbsp honey

2 tbsp raw sugar

4 tbsp sweet almond oil or other base oil

1 tbsp ground lavender flowers

4-5 drops of essential oil of your choice, optional

Mix all the ingredients together until well combined and store in the fridge in an airtight container.

JUICEMAN TIP
Coffee granules work really well too. Use instead of the almond pulp.

QUICK AND EASY BODY SCRUB

There are many things you can do with your leftover pulp, but these body scrubs are a favourite with the missus. Get this bad boy all over you . . . scrub scrub scrub.

50g raw almond pulp or other nut pulp (the grittier the better)

125ml cold-pressed sweet almond oil

1 tbsp raw sugar

the zest of 1 lemon

Stir all the ingredients together until well combined. Store in an airtight container in the fridge.

To use, simply scrub over your body and rinse with water. It will leave you glowing.

JUICEMAN TIP
You can add a few drops of essential oil of your choice for extra fragrance. I particularly like rose oil.

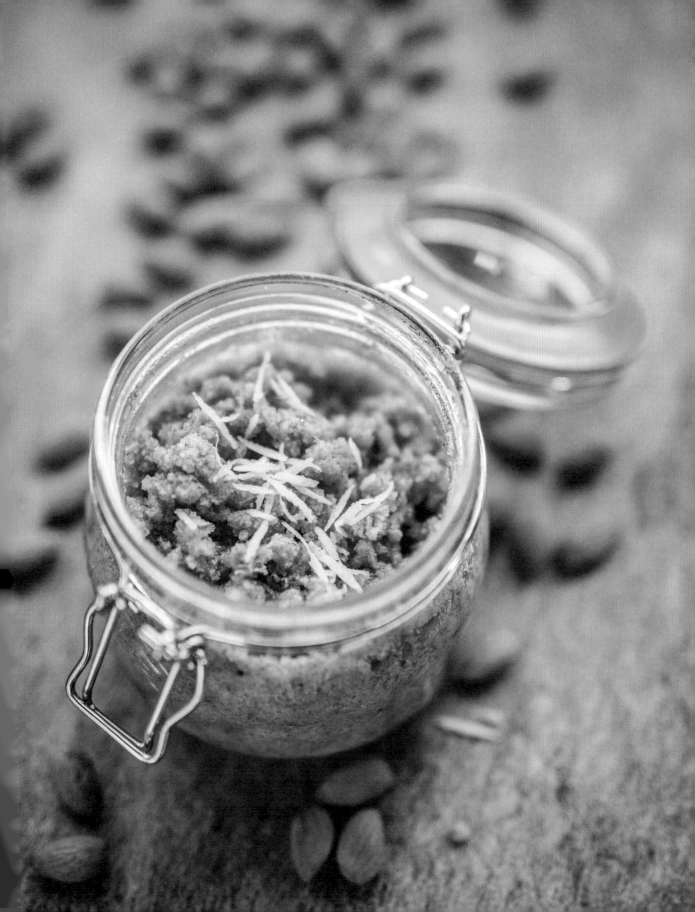

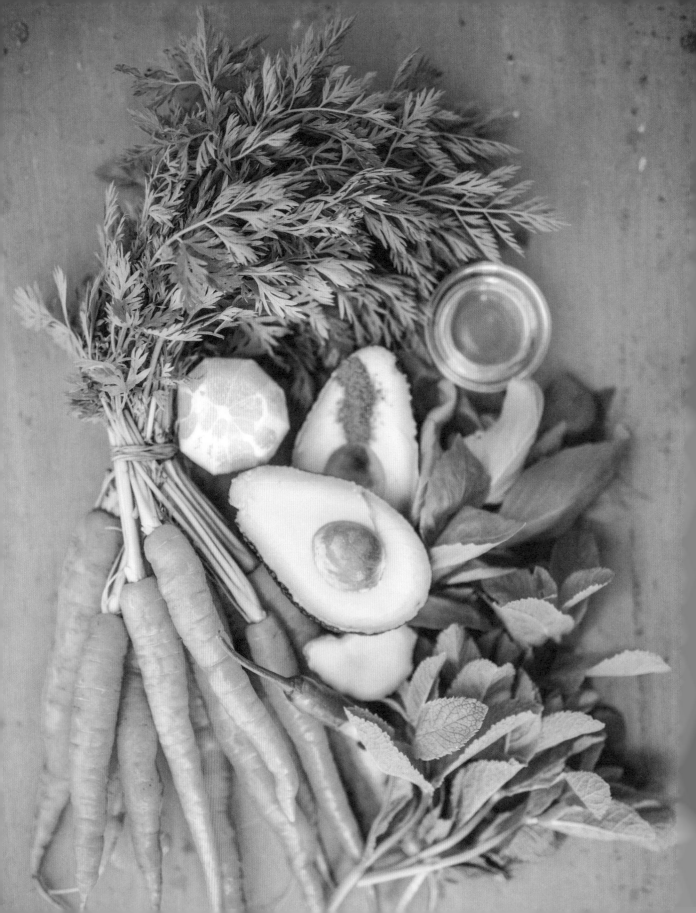

CLEANSE

Fasting is one of the oldest ways of encouraging the human body to heal and naturally rid itself of toxins. On average, we take 18 hours to process each piece of food that we consume. If you consider the fact that we eat three meals a day, and often snack in between, our bodies therefore never stop working.

Over time, toxins build up and coat the internal system, creating an acidic pH, whereas the human body requires an alkaline pH. The western diet, heavy in meat and dairy products, contributes to this build-up. If your colon and digestive system is coated in waste, your body will only be able to absorb a small percentage of the 'good stuff' you consume.

Fasting with juice aids the detoxification process while still ensuring that you get all the necessary nutrition and goodness. The body doesn't need to work hard to digest juice because all the fibre is removed in the juicing process. For the duration of your cleanse, your digestive system will therefore be able to rest and your body can focus on the other things it needs to do, like healing.

Make the changes now and reap the rewards!

A NEED TO REBOOT

I started cleansing as I was beginning to feel the wear and tear of living a fast-paced life, working and travelling a lot while trying to enjoy myself too. I wanted to refresh my body and mind and take some time out to heal. When I did my very first cleanse, a patch of eczema I had had for years just disappeared and has never come back. My skin looks and feels so much better and my eyes are brighter and any dark circles always disappear during a cleanse. I do one at least 5 times a year. You can choose how many days you would like to do, but the longer you do, the more benefits you tend to feel. That said, it is still an achievement to do a one-day cleanse. It's your personal decision.

If you are in any doubt about your health and whether it would suit you to do a cleanse then I suggest that you speak to your doctor about it.

Below is a testimonial from one of our Juiceman cleanse customers that really shows how beneficial juice cleansing can be.

'Being the CEO of an organisation, full-time mum and wife takes its toll. I travel all over the world and spend much of my time at conferences, where good food and great wine are in abundance, so it's no surprise that keeping my weight down has always been a challenge. Over the last few years, though, I had also noticed my lack of energy, increasing muzzy heads and overwhelming sense of exhaustion that would hit every afternoon. It was after a two-week holiday in the Caribbean that I realized that resting had not improved these symptoms and so I turned to a juice cleanse for my first ever detox.

'I found seven consecutive days in my diary when I wasn't invited to some corporate lunch or dinner that I couldn't get out of. I had weaned myself off caffeine over the summer holiday, but I was still out drinking wine the night before I started my detox. I promised myself that I would give it one week of my life and then on the eighth day I would have a supper of steak, triple-cooked chips and Chablis to celebrate. I'm the sort of person that is in 110 per cent or not in it at all, so I knew that I could do it having made the commitment. Then the greatest thing happened . . .

'I expected to feel hungry but I didn't. The first couple of days were easy (it was strange not sitting down to eat with the family in the evening but actually it was quite liberating). It was also strange not thinking about what to cook for dinner. I realized that I eat purely for pleasure. My days would be cheered up by the thought of what delicious dish I would consume in the evening, but I felt really free not having to think about that and I started to think about other nice things I could do, like having a long hot soak in the bath.

'There was a moment on day four when a colleague was taking a bite out of a ham salad roll and I could have snatched it right out of her hands – but I just took a few sips of my juice and the feeling subsided. At this point I started to crave a Cobb salad. I was dreaming of vegetables and salad – no dressing, just crisp, fresh ingredients. However, I also felt tired and sluggish and my head was muzzy again so I went to bed early that night.

'On day five I woke up early, refreshed and full of energy. For the first time in ages I jumped, rather than dragged, myself out of bed and I bounced down the stairs, rather than shuffled! My energy levels matched my five-year-old's that morning and it was a great feeling. My concentration improved at work too and my thinking became clearer.

'At the end of the cleanse, my husband cooked triple-cooked chips but with salmon as the thought of red meat just felt too heavy. I had four or five chips and a small piece of salmon and that was enough. The thought of wine made my nose curl and when I sipped it, yuk, it was like the first time I ever tried wine!

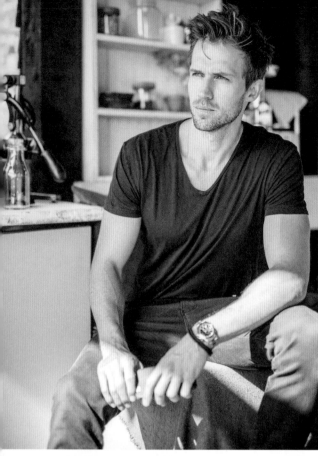

'I have continued to juice and follow a clean lifestyle ever since. I think my system, or at least my palate, has been reset because all of those things like red meat, pasta, wine and chocolate that I used to crave, I'm not bothered about any more. I wish I had done a before and after of my figure and of the inside of my fridge – they both look completely different now! Most importantly though, I feel great, I sleep well and I'm full of enough energy to work and play. I lost eleven pounds in seven days and have now gone on to lose two stone and I feel in the best shape of my life, inside and out.' Simone Buckley.

PRE-CLEANSE ADVICE

The Day Before:

Remove all caffeine, alcohol, dairy and processed foods from your diet. If you are a smoker, you would ideally stop during the cleanse to get the best results. If not, try to cut down – it may even be the catalyst to giving up completely! Today is the perfect day to get some fresh, preferably organic, food to eat. Try and spend your day eating whole fruit, salads, soups and steamed vegetables. If you must eat meat, stick to chicken or have fish instead. The more effort you put into this day the more it will help with the overall cleanse. Do not worry about the thought of having no food and don't eat more than usual to make sure you have enough calories – your juice cleanse will provide you with everything you need in the days to follow. Try to consume your last meal by 6pm or 7pm so that you can get a deeper, more beneficial cleanse in the first day. Also, now is a good time to get your cool bag together if you are going to be out all day. A standard cool bag or cool box, such as you would use on a picnic, complete with ice blocks, should be sufficient. Your juices

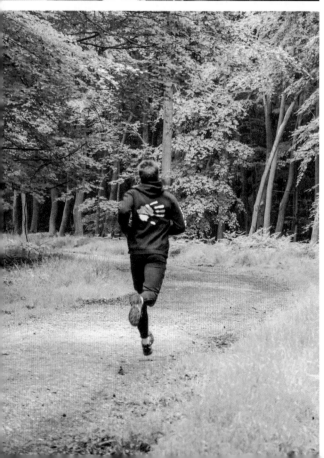

need to be kept refrigerated at all times; failing to do so may damage the product and make it inedible.

It is a good idea to try and plan your days so you allow for enough rest and detox-boosting activities such as:

Exercise – if this is your first cleanse I would do something light and avoid heavy cardio. Walking, yoga (if there's one thing you should do, it's stretch) and light circuits are a good start. If you are an experienced cleanser, you should be able to carry on as normal. One tip is that you will always have optimum energy 30 minutes after your juice so this is a good time to exercise. Also, try and get it done in the morning as you may be more tired between 4pm and 8pm.

Massage – if you can, book yourself in for a deep-tissue massage in order to help your body dispel toxins and increase blood flow.

Sauna and steam – a great way to encourage and speed up the detox. By sweating you are releasing toxins. Make sure you rehydrate after.

Body brush – this will help to eliminate toxins. Always remember to brush towards the heart.

Take a hot salt bath – again, this will help to flush away the toxins. Take some time out for this each evening and you will reap the rewards.

Colonics – everyone should be open minded about this as it's a truly brilliant way to clean your digestive system so your body can absorb all the nutrients properly. If this is not for you, then some sachets of Colosan will encourage bowel movement while cleansing. If you are happy to go ahead with a colonic then try to have one the night before you start or the morning of the first day and then another the morning after you finish.

Sleep and rest – if possible, try and grab a cat nap in the afternoon and make sure you get an early night as sleeping will aid your body's repairing process.

Activated charcoal – I love this stuff. It is a great way to draw out all the toxins your body is holding on to. Simply add a teaspoon to 300ml of mineral water, and add some lemon and maple syrup for a better taste, if you like. Doing this twice daily during your cleanse will help the detoxing process.

Before you go to bed take a selfie and record measurements and weight as a point of comparison.

POST-CLEANSE ADVICE

It is important to ease yourself out of a cleanse the way you eased yourself in. I suggest a green smoothie for breakfast and a light salad for lunch and dinner. Hopefully, you will feel so good that you will only want to eat clean nutritious food. I strongly advise that you avoid alcohol and caffeine for at least 24 hours. I once had a client who had a cappuccino immediately after finishing his cleanse and felt so sick that he never drank coffee again. Bad move, but perhaps a good outcome!

THE PROGRAMME

THE ESSENTIAL CLEANSE

Your essential shopping list contains everything you need to get started. This is per day, so simply multiply the ingredients by the number of days you're cleansing for.

2 ½ lemons
1 lime
3 green apples
1 red apple
1 pear
½ a pink grapefruit
4 celery sticks
1 cucumber
a handful of kale leaves
¼ of a fennel bulb
3 carrots
½ a sweet potato
1 beetroot
1 yellow beetroot
9cm piece of fresh root ginger
2.5cm piece of fresh root turmeric
a small handful of mint leaves

Wake Up	Morning Shot (p.116)
7am	All Hail Kale (p.28)
11am	Beet Box (p.36)
2pm	Cool As Cucumber (p.46)
5pm	Ultimate OJ (p.51)
8pm	Green Love (p.60)

THE SUPER CLEANSE ... FOR THOSE OF YOU WANTING A DEEPER DETOX

Your super shopping list contains everything you need to get started. This is per day, so simply multiply the ingredients by the number of days you're cleansing for.

3 lemons
1 orange
½ a lime
1 apple
2 pears
a handful of grapes
1 rhubarb stick (if seasonal)
¼ of a pineapple
2 ¼ cucumbers
8 celery sticks
a large handful of kale leaves
1 chard leaf
½ a head of pak choi
2 carrots
½ a courgette
¼ of a fennel bulb
a handful of spinach leaves
12cm piece of fresh root ginger
2.5cm piece of fresh root turmeric
a pinch of cayenne pepper
a few leaves of fresh rosemary
a bunch of coriander
2.5cm slice of lemongrass
a small bunch of parsley
8 drops of echinacea
1 tsp MSM powder
1 tsp aloe vera juice

Wake Up	The Healer (p.122)
7am	Green Love (p.60)
11am	Winter Cold Kicker (p.62)
2pm	Mean Green (p.42)
5pm	Green Rocket (p.42)
8pm	Green Roots (p.43)

FREEZE WITH EASE

Chopped fruit is brilliant for speeding up your juice- and smoothie-making process. As well as this, consider making a big batch of juice, nut milk or shots to freeze as ice lollies and ice cubes.

This is a great way to plan ahead and by buying your produce in bulk, you'll get more value for your money.

Here are some of my favourite recipes to freeze, but in all honesty, you can freeze anything – from straight kale juice to cashew milk.

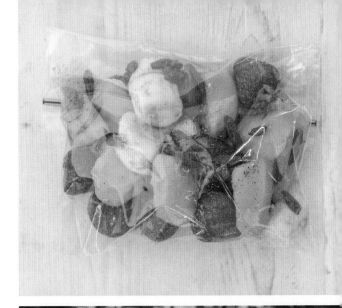

ICE CUBES

1 Cool as a Cucumber – a great addition to a gin and tonic (p.46)

2 Morning Shot – enjoy in warm water first thing in the morning (p.116)

3 Deep Green – add some extra green goodness to your green smoothie (p.35)

4 Almond Milk – perfect for adding to smoothies (p.141)

5 100% turmeric – great to add to any juice or smoothie and a quick way to make Turmeric Milk when blitzed with nut milk

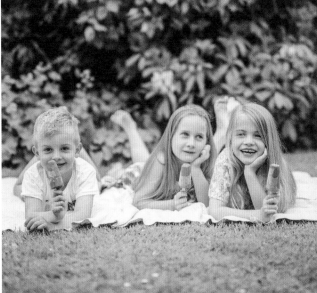

ICE LOLLIES

1 PPG (p.45)

2 Ultimate OJ (p.51)

3 Orange Healer (p.34)

4 Watermelon Cooler (p.26)

5 Juiceman Daiquiri (p.188)

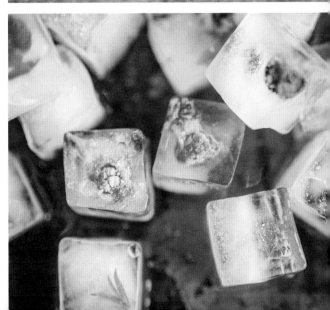

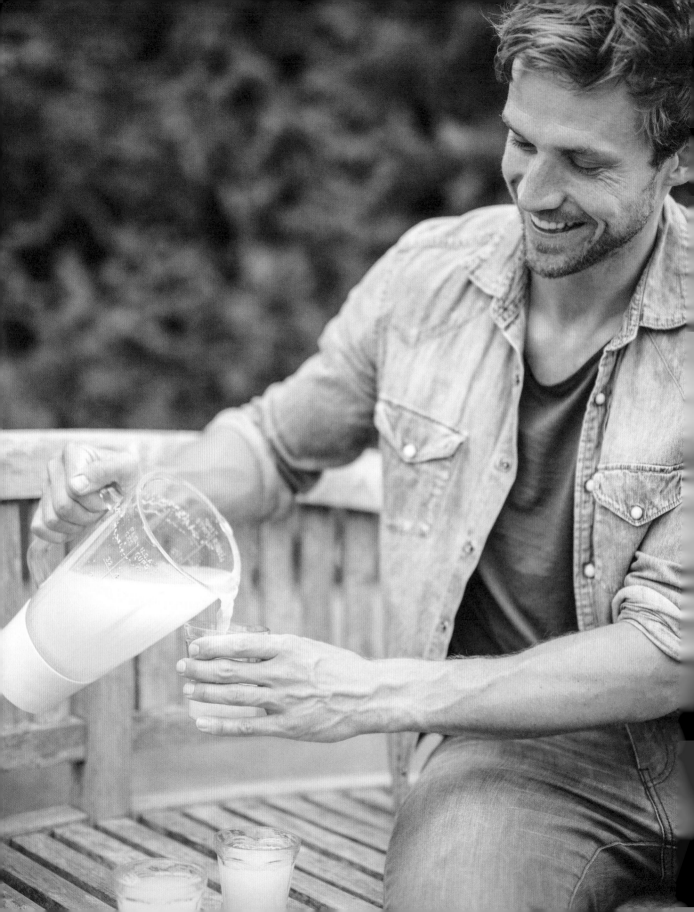

Q&A

Why is juicing supposedly more effective for nutrient absorption versus actually eating the solid fruit and vegetables?

It's not, it is just a much easier and quicker way to get nutrients into your body. If you want to get the best results, it is important to incorporate a fat into your juices, whether it's a teaspoon of coconut oil or hemp oil, half an avocado or just some raw nuts. Juicing is a way to support a healthier lifestyle, not a way to replace eating.

My dentist yells at me for drinking too many smoothies (acid erosion of the teeth). Is there anything else besides drinking through a straw that I can do to help this?

The more citrus-based juices and smoothies, especially shots, can affect the enamel of your teeth (depending on their condition). I've actually never had this problem, but the advice I would give is to avoid brushing your teeth straight after a drink, even your morning lemon and ginger tea, as this could push the acid deeper into the enamel.

Does adding protein powder to a smoothie lessen the blood sugar spike?

Yes, protein is important to prevent the blood sugar spikes which make you feel weak and dizzy. You can add extra protein to your smoothie by including soaked nuts and seeds, protein powder or spirulina. You can also add fibre in the form of flaxseeds, chia seeds, rolled oats, or wheat germ to slow down the absorption of glucose.

Whenever I try to bulk out my smoothies with ice cubes, the result falls flat. Help!

This can be a problem, depending on your blender. Ice takes a few seconds to mix in. If you are unable to get the mix going, add some liquid and give it a shake.

Can I really get full from a juice?

Absolutely, if it's a dense green one. One of the key things is to chew your juice and take your time. This way your body accepts it as food and it's easier to digest. Due to the lack of fibre in a juice, a smoothie will be a more filling option though.

Is it safe to juice every day?

There are no doubt many opinions on this, but my view is yes, definitely. I think everyone is different and their nutritional needs will vary. I have juiced every day for over ten years and believe it's the reason why I feel strong and healthy. You should vary what you juice and support it with a healthy diet and exercise. It is definitely not a wonder cure but it's a healthy habit that provides great nutritional benefits.

Do I need to spend a lot of money on a juicer? How do I choose one?

Generally, the rule is that the more you spend, the better-quality machine you get. My Omega and Vitamix juicers are still going strong after five years – and they've had to endure a lot of use. I also think it's important to understand the yield aspect of a juicer. With a low rpm cold-press mechanism you can get a good 10 per cent yield, especially off leafy green veg. So if you juice every day, it will pay for itself against a cheaper high-speed juicer.

There seem to be many different smoothie makers and juicers out there. What are the best ones?

Here are my recommendations (cheapest first):

Juicers:	Blenders:
Omega Vert	NutriBullet
Breville	Vitamix
Philips	Ninja

Does it tend to be the more expensive the better?

With juicers, I would say yes. They produce better quality juice and yield, which will be more economical on your annual produce spend. With blenders, I feel the NutriBullet provides a great simple solution. The reason to purchase a Vitamix is for larger volume per use and a greater variety of uses. One thing I will say is that a Vitamix will never be as good as a food processor at making nut butters, dips, cake mixtures, etc. due to the surface size of the blade and base of jug.

Can I swap a meal for a juice?

Yes, absolutely. Just not every meal, unless you are specifically cleansing. I have gone seven days on just juice and felt amazing, but you need the right preparation. In general, if you have had a big breakfast and lunch you will probably sleep better on a light dinner, which could be a green juice or smoothie. I for one consider 1kg of fresh vegetables in a juice a better meal than a pizza.

What's the best juice for a detox?

Ones that are low in fruit content and high in green veg, celery, aloe vera: ingredients that will cleanse you and replenish your system. Check out the Cleanse section on pages 200–205.

Is there really too much sugar in fruit and natural fruit juice?

Everything in moderation! There is no hiding that there is sugar in fruit and fruit juices. But as long as you're not consuming large amounts of them and you're energetic and active enough, the sugar shouldn't be a problem for you. Our bodies will convert it to energy. Otherwise it can be stored as fat. A lot has been said about the high sugar content of juices and smoothies and that they're not as good for us as we think. Many commercial drinks are indeed overloaded with sweet-tasting ingredients, can be highly processed and made with heat-inducing cooking methods. However, making fresh juices and smoothies at home is a whole different ball game.

Can I put yogurt in a smoothie – or will that undo all my hard work?

It depends on what you are looking for and what kind of yogurt. There is nothing wrong with a treat and personally I love coconut yogurt or kefir in a smoothie.

Ditto juice . . . sometimes I add shop-bought juice to the blended fruit. Am I just pouring sugary badness into my healthy drink? Are there certain types of juice I should avoid?

YES! This is a Juiceman no-no. Unless we are talking cold-pressed juice, coconut water or nut milk. Heat-pasteurized juices have effectively been cooked and many have had sugar added, which means you are indeed ruining your good work.

What's the best drink to give you energy?

Ingredients like chilli and ginger are great for kick-starting your system and metabolism. My go-to if I'm having a sluggish start to the day is a green smoothie with a few dates and a scoop of maca powder for an added kick. If you are really in need of some energy, add yerba maté tea to your drink.

What's the best drink after a workout?

One that is hydrating, so look out for one containing a high percentage of cucumber or coconut, for example. Protein is key to keeping strong and maintaining or building muscle mass.

What's the best drink to help calm a stomach?

Ginger is great to settle your stomach and combat nausea. Sugar is also good, so drinks containing pineapple or apple, for instance. If it's related to digestive issues, then I would try taking a shot of live apple cider vinegar daily before each meal to help with your digestion.

What should be the ratio of vegetables to fruit in a juice or smoothie?

Ideally 20 per cent fruit to 80 per cent veg. Saying that, there is nothing wrong with an all-fruit juice – as long as you're not drinking massive amounts of it. I typically like to break my juices up as 80 per cent veg (50 per cent leafy greens and herbs), 15 per cent fruit and 5 per cent citrus and spice. Layer spinach in between fruit or use high-water-content veg like cucumbers or carrots.

What time of day do you have your smoothie/juice?

I tend to start my day with a juice and then have a smoothie after a workout or as a meal replacement in the evening. If I'm feeling a bit flat and run-down, I will have a couple of shots too.

Do you tend to have a smoothie instead of a meal and a juice with a meal?

Yes, exactly. If I'm having prawn spaghetti or scrambled eggs and avocado on toast there is nothing better than a green juice to provide extra nutrients.

What are the best ingredients for an energy boost?

Dates
Maca powder
Raw cacao
Yerba maté

What are good detoxing ingredients?

Leafy greens
Lemon
Spirulina
Chlorella
Celery

If you're having a smoothie for breakfast, can you get enough protein from just fruits and vegetables or should you add a protein powder?

Definitely add protein. There is a myth around protein being more for men and people wanting to bulk out. In fact, good levels of protein make your body better at burning fat.

What are your thoughts on adding powders such as spirulina to juices and smoothies?

Spirulina is such an amazing ingredient and top of the chain in terms of phytonutrients and minerals. It contains 15 times more calcium than milk. It can be quite overpowering, though, so I recommend it in smoothies more than juices as you can hide the taste. Trying to put powders into juices is tough.

What are your top tips for a juice cleanse?

Prep, prep and prep. Eliminating your vices (alcohol, coffee, red meat, etc.) at least 24 hours prior to a cleanse makes a huge difference. Also adopting a more vegan raw diet is a great way to maximise the goodness. Try to get your body ready the day before by having a chia pot with fruit for breakfast, soup or smoothie for lunch and a salad for dinner. This way your body will start by making adjustments.

Should you exercise while doing a cleanse?

It's personal preference, but it's great to get your metabolism going to help expel toxins. This can be anything from undertaking a light gym session or some yoga, to going for a jog. I once ran five miles each day on a five-day cleanse and found it was easy. The key things I recommend are at least eight hours sleep, hot salt baths and plenty of water. If you can get a colonic or sauna/steam, then even better.

How long can you keep juices in the fridge after you've made them?

If you use a low rpm cold-press juicer, I would say 24 to 48 hours. But they're always best fresh. Any high rpm juicer will cause heat friction, meaning that the juice starts to oxidize straight away and effectively go off. Drink these juices immediately. At Juiceman, we use the freshest veg and fruit and make the juices in a cold room to ensure the best unpasteurized juice possible. Even taking into account those procedures, I always say the sooner you drink it the better.

How can you make a juice actually fill you up until lunch?

Loading it full of green veg will help. Ultimately I recommend smoothies more as meal replacements because they have fibre in them. A lot depends on your goal. If you want to lose weight, then low-fibre juices will be more effective as a meal replacement.

Is it worth buying a NutriBullet?

Yes, I absolutely love the NutriBullet and think it's already responsible for a huge shift in attitudes towards healthy eating. The fact that it is so powerful and well priced means it's a great starter tool. There is also little waste and they're very easy to clean.

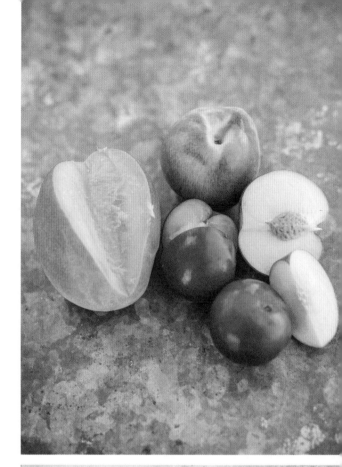

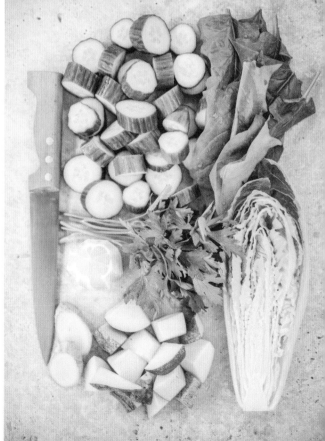

Can a peanut butter smoothie ever be healthy? (There's a lot riding on this question. I hope the answer is yes!)

Peanuts are funny ones as there are two sides to them. The less commercial raw and unsalted ones are a great source of magnesium, folate, vitamin E, copper, arginine and fibre. The downside is that they are also loaded with fats – even though they are healthy fats – so watch your intake. If you're using the roasted and salted peanuts like the ones you get in the pub then the answer is definitely no!

What's the best fruit juice or smoothie option which isn't so high in sugar?

Any that is vegetable-based or at least 70 per cent green vegetables. Also watermelon is a great option because of its high water content.

What's your favourite combination for a smoothie or juice?

Kale, pineapple, cucumber, lime, celery, ginger and coriander for a juice. For a smoothie, I like Thai flavours. If it's a smoothie I will often add my faves: coconut butter, hemp seeds, cinnamon and a date with some almond milk or water.

What's your favourite smoothie ingredient?

Activated barley and spirulina for their health properties. For sheer pleasure, cashew butter and coconut butter!

What's a great pre- or post-workout smoothie?

Chocolate Power Shake (p.91) and Pink Power Shake (p.92) are great . . .

When doing a juice cleanse should you be careful how much fruit is in the juices?

Absolutely, but it's also about getting through it the first time so I recommend keeping it palatable on your first go. I also recommend setting yourself a realistic target. Try for 36 hours or 2 days but be prepared to extend if you're feeling comfortable. Some people find it easy and some not.

Are all juicing machines fiendishly hard to clean?

No, not at all. The newer models are becoming a lot easier to clean. I always recommend putting water through your machine after each time you use it and then soaking all parts in hot soapy water at the end of the day.

Is it true that juicing leeks and garlic in high quantities can cause stomach upsets?

Probably. I wouldn't recommend eating high volumes of raw garlic and leeks either. My first cleanse involved a juice with raw garlic and onions and it is still my least favourite juice ever. I recommend things like garlic to be put in a shot if you are going to use them.

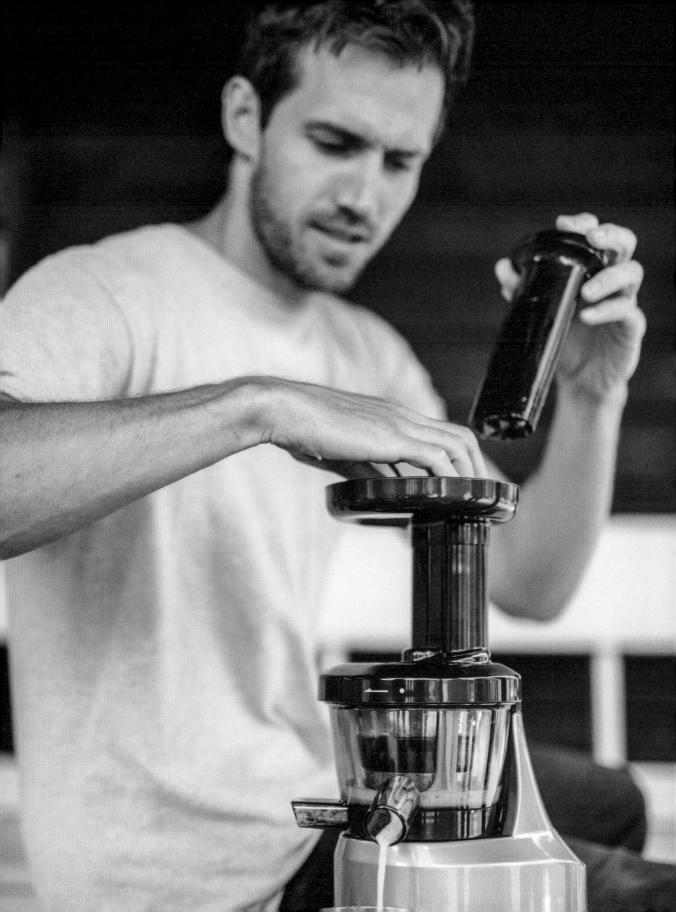

DR JUICE

COLD AND FLU / IMMUNITY BOOST

A strong immune system is essential for maintaining good health and wellbeing. Since adapting my diet to include raw organic food, juices and smoothies, I've been surprised at how I'm able to avoid getting sick and don't suffer from general fatigue.

Turn to these recipes when you feel the initial signs of a cold or flu coming on. They will help your body to fight it off while keeping you feeling energized. Make sure you have a high intake of vitamin C and incorporate Echinacea, apple cider vinegar, turmeric and ginger in your juices and smoothies. There are some great shots here for clearing your sinuses too.

Juiceman recommends
Echinacea
Lemon
Orange
Ginger
Turmeric
Oregano oil
Parsley
Goji berries
Chaga mushroom

Juices: The Original (p.25)
Ultimate OJ (p.51)
Love it Spicy Green (p.63)
Winter Cold Kicker (p.62)

Smoothies: Immunity Boost (p.75)
Flu Jab (p.109)

Shots: Raw Heat (p.116)
Get Well (p.113)
Fire Ball (p.122)

Teas: Hot Cider Healer (p.127)

ALKALISING

Research shows that keeping the body's pH alkaline (our optimum pH is around 7.4) increases vitality and prevents illness. You can buy a test kit and measure your level quite easily. Great ingredients for encouraging alkalinity are superfoods such as spirulina and chlorella. Strangely enough, some highly acidic ingredients also create an alkaline environment in the body, such as apple cider vinegar and citrus fruits such as lemon and lime.

Juiceman recommends
Lemon
Lime
Spirulina
Chlorella
Kale
Cucumber
Celery
Broccoli
Cabbage
Apple cider vinegar

Juices: Cool as a Cucumber (p.46)
Mean Green (p.42)
Love it Spicy Green (p.63)
Alkalise (p.64)

Smoothies: Supermum (p.81)
Green Warrior (p.90)
The Royal Green (p.100)

Shots: Morning Shot (p.116)

DETOXIFYING

We are exposed to harmful toxins daily – even the chemicals in household cleaning products and pharmaceutical drugs contribute towards toxicity within the body and can overburden our system. This section is about encouraging the release and removal of toxins. To help with this, drink a pint of water first thing in the morning to flush the system. You could even try adding some activated charcoal to help draw out the toxins.

Juiceman recommends
E3Live
Chlorella
Spirulina
Wheatgrass
Probiotics
Activated charcoal
Psyllium husks

Juices: Thai Green (p.53)
Green Glow (p.59)
Deep Green (p.35)

Smoothies: Skin Food (p.34)
Green Love (p.60)

Shot: Activated Charcoal Tonic (p.120)

Teas: Teatox (p.134)

DIGESTION

Our gut is our 'second brain' and the key to good health. And yet it is often abused. Having had first hand experience of a gut infection, I strongly recommend that you pay it due attention. There are many ways to help maintain a healthy digestive system – from making sure you chew your food properly to juice cleansing and having a good probiotic programme. My tip is to always make sure you do a full probiotic course after any antibiotic prescription.

Juiceman recommends
Perm A vite
Chia seeds
Psyllium husk
Aloe vera
L-Glutamine
Cayenne pepper
Cinnamon
Apple cider vinegar
Probiotics (I recommend Symprove)

Juices: Pink Healer (p.40)
Green Hero (p.43)

Smoothies: Supermum (p.81)
Green Bangkok (p.97)

Shots: Tummy Tuck (p.116)

Tea: Moroccan Mint Tea (p.133)

PRE WORKOUT

Depending on what kind of workout you're undertaking and what your goals are, there are some things to consider when it comes to fuelling your body. If you are looking to burn fat, focus on cardio exercise first thing in the morning while you're in a fasted state – but nothing too strenuous: a slow jog for an hour or a yoga or Pilates session are good options. If you are looking to maintain or increase muscle mass, it's important to fuel your workout. Heavy sessions will require both carbs and protein. I will have a small protein shake 30–60 minutes before training and snack on things like dates and bananas. Yerba maté tea is a great way to kick-start your energy. It will give you a caffeine boost. Powders such as activated barley, lucuma and maca are great for slow-release energy.

Juiceman recommends
Raw honey
Yerba maté
Chia seeds
Medjool dates
Activated barley
Maca
Lucuma
Cacao nibs
Cashew nuts
Banana
Mango
Cayenne pepper
Ginseng

Juices: Beet Box (p.36)
The J5 (p.46)
Smoothies: Tropical Thunder (p.96)
Fire-Starter (p.76)
Pick-Me-Up (p.96)
The Incredibles (p.84)
Hurricane (p.91)
Mango Punch (p.107)
Shots: Morning Shot (p.116)
Smoothie Bowls:
Green Giant Breakfast Bowl (p.162)

RECOVERY/POST WORKOUT

Recovery is all about providing your body with the right nutrients to refuel and repair. Staying well hydrated throughout the day and sleeping efficiently at night are also essential. A protein smoothie after a workout will help the body repair and build muscle tissue – L-Glutamine and protein powder are brilliant for this. Including chia seeds and shelled hemp will also provide good levels of omega-3 and -6. If you are looking to burn fat, I'd advise having green juice or a yerba maté tea for energy. Add turmeric for its anti-inflammatory properties. Your body continues to burn fat even after you've finished working out, so wait twenty minutes or so before refueling if this is your aim.

Juiceman recommends
Chia seeds
Hemp seeds
Natural protein powder
Activated whey
Almonds
Glucosamine
Turmeric
Activated barley
L-Glutamine
E3-Live
Essential fatty acids
Branch chain amino acids
Coconut oil

Juices: Wimbledon Winner (p.48)
Pineappleade (p.66)
Smoothies: Hurricane (p.91)
Green Warrior (p.90)
Be Good to Yourself (p.105)
Pink Power Shake (p.92)
Chocolate Power Shake (p.91)
Shots: Yoga Shot (p.118)

BEAUTY

Beauty comes from within, and this applies to your health too. Nowadays, we're just not getting enough of the vitamins, oils and minerals that our bodies need for maintaining optimum health. Healthy-looking hair, skin and nails all require good levels of essential fatty acids and vitamins C, B, K2 and D. Minerals such as silica, niacin, zinc and sulphur are important too. My wife swears by the supplement MSM – it is a natural source of sulphur and can help improve the elasticity of skin and hair.

Juiceman recommends
MSM
Chia seeds
Deer antler extract
Aloe vera
Coconut oil
Cashew nuts
Cucumber
Hemp seeds
Macadamia nuts
Pumpkin seeds
Turmeric
Green leafy veg – kale, chard, etc

Juices: Cool as a Cucumber (p.46)
Skin Food (p.34)
Green Glow (p.59)
Green Ninja (p.46)

Smoothies: Skin Love (p.72)
Taylor's Favourite Tipple (p.82)
Blueberry Facial (p.84)
The Secret Smoothie (p.99)

Shots: Skin Shot (p.115)

Smoothie Bowls: Forever Young (p.162)

WEIGHT LOSS

Start by assessing your diet and daily routine. Are you eating too many processed foods? Biscuits, sweets and crisps are one of the biggest causes of weight gain. The first thing to do is cut all of these out of your diet. Also try to start your day with 1 litre of mineral water to encourage the cleansing process. You could even try a 3-, 5- or 7-day juice cleanse. At Juiceman we have had some amazing results with our juice cleanses – one client lost 11 lbs in 7 days! If you are looking for low-calorie juices, stick to the green juices with little or no fruit.

There are some ingredients that speed up metabolism and digestion, such as yerba maté tea and cayenne pepper. Fruit and veg with a high water content, such as cucumber and watermelon, are healthy low-calorie options. The smoothies below can also be used as meal replacements.

Juiceman recommends
Yerba maté
Grapefruit
Melon
Watermelon
Cucumber

Juices: Skinny Jeans (p.54)
Watermelon Cooler (p.26)

Smoothies: Diet Smoothie (p.97)
Green Warrior (p.90)
Green Bangkok (p.97)

Shots: Tummy Tuck (p.116)
Fireball (p.122)
Activated Charcoal Tonic (p.120)

Teas: Hot Cider Healer (p.127)

HEALING

Some of my favourite healing superfoods are: turmeric, which boasts some unbelievable cancer-fighting properties; apple cider vinegar, which is one of the oldest tonics and has been used for a wide range of medicinal purposes – both as an internal medicine and as a topical cure; and medicinal mushrooms, which are widely considered to be a wonder cure in Asia. They have unparalleled amounts of antioxidants and healing benefits. If I'm in need of a boost, I will put a teaspoon in my smoothie twice a day and feel like Superman.

Juiceman recommends
Turmeric
Apple cider vinegar
Chaga mushroom
Reishi mushroom
Manuka honey
Aloe vera
MSM
L-Glutamine
Hemp oil
E3Live and other algae, such as spirulina
Argan oil

Juices: Ultimate OJ (p.51)
Green Rocket (p.42)
Green Hero (p.43)
Smoothies: Mango Magic (p.88)
The Royal Green (p.100)
Be Good to Yourself (p.105)
Shots: SOS (p.116)
The Healer (p.122)
Last Resort (p.123)
Teas: Hot Cider Healer (p.127)

STRESS

Physical and mental stress can wreak havoc on your health. Good nutrition and sufficient sleep are incredibly important in combatting stress. Listen to your body. When you feel tired, try to rest – don't be a hero and battle through it. This section suggests foods to combine to help your body and mind relax.

Juiceman recommends
Cashew nuts
Cacao nibs
Chamomile
Blueberries
Oranges
Walnuts
Almonds
Spinach
E3Live
Chlorella
Ginseng

Juices: Orange Healer (p.34)
Smoothies: Chocolate Rebel (p.86)
Blueberry Facial (p.84)
The Royal Green (p.100)
Hurricane (p.91)
Nut milks: Almond milk (p.141)
Cashew Milk (p.142)

STOCKISTS AND SUPPLIERS

JUICERS AND BLENDERS

JUICELAND
www.juiceland.com

JOHN LEWIS
www.johnlewis.com

ARGOS
www.argos.com

HUROM
www.huromuk.com

ORGANIC FOODS, NATURAL PRODUCTS AND HEALTH SUPPLEMENTS

JUICEMAN
Cold Pressed Juice
www.juiceman.co

DAYLESFORD
Home grown and locally sourced
organic produce
www.daylesford.com

ABEL & COLE
Organic food delivery
www.abelandcole.co.uk

EVOLUTION ORGANICS
General health store
www.evolutionorganics.co.uk

RED23
Online health store
www.red23.com

AS NATURE INTENDED
General health store
www.asnatureintended.uk.com

BIONA
www.biona.co.uk

RAW HEALTH
www.rawhealth.uk.com

DR MERCOLA
Supplements and vitamins
www.mercola.com

ARTISANA ORGANICS
Nut butters and coconut oil
www.artisanaorganics.com

THE RAW HONEY SHOP
www.therawhoneyshop.com

MIGHTY BEE
Coconut water
www.mightybee.com

SUNWARRIOR
Vegan protein powders
www.sunwarrior.com

JING TEA
www.jingtea.com

DRAGON HERBS
Exotic herbs and tonics
www.dragonherbs.com

LIFORME
Yoga mats
www.liforme.com

RESTAURANTS AND JUICE BARS

LONDON
Ottolenghi www.ottolenghi.co.uk
The Electric Diner www.theelectricdiner.com
Nama www.namafoods.com
Granger & Co www.grangerandco.com
Wild Food Cafe www.wildfoodcafe.com

LA
Moon Juice www.moonjuiceshop.com
Cafe Gratitude www.cafegratitude.com

NEW YORK
Hu Kitchen www.hukitchen.com
Juice Press www.juicepress.com
The Butcher's Daughter
www.thebutchersdaughter.com
The Fat Radish www.thefatradishnyc.com

INDEX

THANK YOU

First of all, thank you for buying this book. I set out to share my lifestyle in a fun and accessible way and I hope I've achieved that.

Thank you to everyone who has ever bought a Juiceman juice and follows the brand and me on our journey.

There are so many people who have influenced me – from my local greengrocer to talented chefs – that I don't know where to begin. Without the help of everyone, this book would never have happened.

First of all, to my book agent, Rachel Mills, at PFD: thank you for reaching out and making this happen (I know I owe you a yoga mat!).

To the wonderful guys at Penguin who have worked so hard on getting this book out there. To my publisher, Lindsey Evans – you are awesome and thanks for all your creative help and for being very patient. The same goes to Zoe Berville and Sophie Elletson.

To the great team who put the shoot together: Al Richardson for his photographs, Joe Woodhouse and Laurie Hill for the food styling and Emma Lahaye for the props.

To the design team at Smith & Gilmour: Alex, Emma and Zoe.

My motivation is my two beautiful children, Taylor and Jackson. They inspire me to better myself and look at the world as their future.

Thank you to my wonderful wife, Jane. Without your help, often late into the night, I would never have finished this book. Your support and belief means the world to me and keeps me going.

To my mum, who has always showed me that following the crowd is too easy and to think outside the box. Thanks, Mum, for making me pick the veggies every Sunday and teaching me about food and alternative medicine . . . yes, I did listen!

To my dad for all his advice and for keeping me on the right track.

Thank you to the rest of my family: Mark, Sophie, James, Adam, Jack, Uncle Mike, Gran, Karen, Liam and Marina. And the gang: Charlie, Georgia, Lyla, Ethan and Sky.

Thank you to my good friends who are always there for me: Pete, Lou Lou, Andy, Nisse, Matt, Will, Simon, Kevin, Georgia.

A big thank you to Gavin Myall, my manager, for providing some calm in what has been a crazy year.

And lastly to the team at Juiceman for all your hard work and effort to create something special. Here's to a fantastic year in 2016!

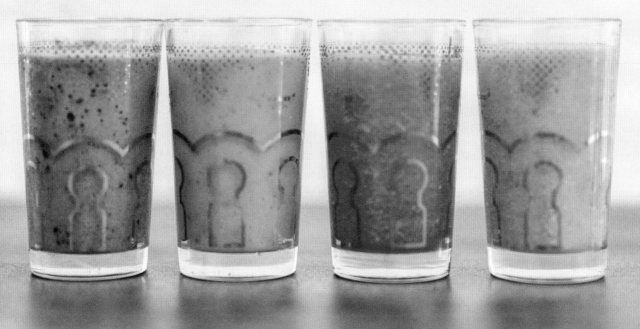

Andrew Cooper is a model and an actor. He has appeared in numerous high-profile print and TV campaigns for brands including Dunhill, Topman, Georgio Armani, Paul Smith and Diet Coke. His love of juicing began at an early age, thanks to his mum, and has since become a way of life and a business venture through his range of Juiceman products. Andrew lives in Buckinghamshire with his wife and two children.

MICHAEL JOSEPH

UK | USA | Canada | Ireland | Australia
India | New Zealand | South Africa

Michael Joseph is part of the Penguin Random House group of companies whose addresses can be found at global.penguinrandomhouse.com.

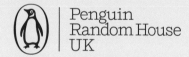
Penguin
Random House
UK

First published 2016
001

Text copyright © Andrew Cooper, 2016
Photographs copyright © Alistair Richardson, 2016

The moral right of the author has been asserted

Design by Smith & Gilmour

Printed and bound in China
A CIP catalogue record for this book is available from the British Library

ISBN: 978-0-718-18305-9

www.greenpenguin.co.uk

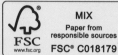